Medical Procedures, Testing and Technology

nova
Medicine & Health
New York

Medical Procedures, Testing and Technology

ELISA: Advances in Research and Applications
Jose Ma. M. Angeles, PhD (Editor)
2022. ISBN: 978-1-68507-500-2 (Hardcover)
2022. ISBN: 978-1-68507-594-1 (eBook)

Principles and Practices of Non-Invasive Mechanical Ventilation Monitoring: From Intensive Care to Home Care
Antonio M. Esquinas (Editor)
2021. ISBN: 978-1-53619-689-4 (Hardcover)
2021. ISBN: 978-1-53619-850-8 (eBook)

The Practice and Principles of Extra-Corporeal Membrane Oxygenation (ECMO)
Michael S. Firstenberg (Editor)
2021. ISBN: 978-1-53618-960-5 (Hardcover)
2021. ISBN: 978-1-53619-093-9 (eBook)

An Introduction to Assistive Technology
Suraj Singh Senjam (Editor)
2020. ISBN: 978-1-53618-935-3 (Hardcover)
2020. ISBN: 978-1-53618-970-4 (eBook)

Testing and Contact Tracing for COVID-19
Ernesto M. Batista (Editor)
2020. ISBN: 978-1-53618-857-8 (Hardcover)
2020. ISBN: 978-1-53618-885-1 (eBook)

More information about this series can be found at
https://novapublishers.com/product-category/series/medical-procedures-testing-and-technology/

Wenli Sun and
Mohamad Hesam Shahrajabian

Various Methods and Novel Techniques

Rapid Molecular Detection of Human, Plant, Genetic, and Microbial Infectious Diseases, Pathogenic Bacteria, and Organisms

nova
Medicine & Health
New York

DOI: https://doi.org/10.52305/CYDP5385

Library of Congress Cataloging-in-Publication Data

ISBN: 978-1-68507-721-1

Published by Nova Science Publishers, Inc. † New York

Contents

Preface[*]

Different isothermal amplification methods are the signal amplification assays, the probe amplification assays, and the target amplification assays. Molecular techniques used for recognition of quinolone resistance consist of the use of various techniques such as polymerase chain reaction fragment length polymorphism, PCR, single-strand conformation polymorphism, nucleotide-sequencing analysis and multiplex allele-specific polymerase chain reaction. Main nucleic acid testing techniques are amplified nucleic acid techniques, microarrays, and non-amplified acid techniques. Non-amplified nucleic acid techniques consist of DNA labeled probes and RNA labeled probes. Molecular methods have considerable benefits for the programmatic management of drug resistance. The PCR-based methods have high sensitivity and specificity, but several molecular tests which employ non-PCR-based methods are developed for rapid detection of RNA such as isothermal nucleic acid amplification like loop mediated isothermal amplification and nucleic acid sequence-based amplification. The most notable methods which can be used to detect pathogens are biochemical assays, immunological assays and polymerase chain reaction (PCR)-based testing of bacterial nucleic acids. The reliability and sensitivity of PCR assays depend on DNA quality. The real-time PCR method can be more specific and involves complex processing steps and requires prior sequence data of the specific target gene.

Loop-mediated isothermal amplification (LAMP) is a powerful and specific DNA-based detection method which can be used on-site. LAMP methods can be more specific than qPCR and immunoassays. Loop-mediated isothermal amplification can be used for detection of both DNA and RNA viruses and applies for diagnosis of various important emerging and re-

[*] This work was supported by the National Key R&D Program of China (Research grant 2019YFA0904700)
All authors contributed equally to literature research, writing manuscript, etc.
The authors declare that they have no potential conflicts of interest.

emerging diseases. LAMP rapidly amplifies nucleic acids with high specificity and sensitivity under isothermal conditions. LAMP technology has been widely used for the detection of human pathogenic bacteria, crop pests, pathogenic organisms and components in meat products. The LAMP assay can be used in the field of molecular diagnosis of cancer, identification of genetically modified organisms, detection of food adulteration, eutrophication, food allergens, pesticides, identification of medicinal plants, drug resistance and DNA methylation studies. The LAMP assay can be used for rapid detection of SARS-CoV, MERS-CoV, SARS-CoV-2, influenza, lymphocystis disease virus, swine acute diarrhea syndrome coronavirus, swine vesicular disease virus, classical swine fever virus, infectious bursal disease virus, marek's disease virus, human papillomaviruses, infectious bronchitis virus, Newcastle disease virus, sacbrood virus, beak and feather disease virus, foot-and-mouth disease virus, bovine herpesvirus-1, milk vetch dwarf virus, etc.

PCR is a very sensitive technique which allows rapid amplification of a specific segment of DNA; PCR makes billions of copies of a specific DNA fragment or gene, which allows detection and identification of gene sequences using visual techniques based on size and charge, and modified versions of PCR have allowed quantitative measurements of gene expression with techniques called real-time PCR. The most important limitations of the PCR method consist of: the DNA polymerase used in the PCR reaction being prone to errors, leading to mutations in the fragment generated; the specificity of the generated PCR product being potentially altered by nonspecific binding of the primers to other similar sequences on the template DNA; and the necessity of some prior sequence information to design primers to generate a PCR product in most cases. Contamination or nonspecific priming can lead to false-positive results, and of the most concern is that PCR detects nucleic acids whether or not they come from viable cells.

LAMO is much more sensitive and specific when compared to PCR for detection of viral diseases. Recombinase Polymerase Amplification is a relatively new isothermal methodology for amplifying DNA. Recombinase aided amplification (RAA) assay has been successfully applied in the detection of bacterial and viral pathogens and overcomes the technical difficulties posed by DNA amplification methods because it does not need thermal denaturation of the template and operates at a low and constant temperature.

Wenli Sun
PhD, Associate Professor
Biotechnology Research Institute, Chinese Academy of Agricultural Sciences, Beijing, China

Mohamad Hesam Shahrajabian
PhD, Senior Researcher
Biotechnology Research Institute, Chinese Academy of Agricultural Sciences, Beijing, China

Chapter 1

Introduction

Nuclic acid amplification technologies are used in the field of molecular biology and recombinant DNA technologies which are used as leading methods in detecting and analyzing a small quantity of nucleic acids (Gill and Ghaemi, 2008). PCR is an enzymatic method to produce numerous copies of a gene by separating the two strands of the DNA containing the gene segment, marking its location with a primer, and using a DNA polymerase to assemble a copy alongside each segment and continuously copy the copies (Shen et al., 2020). PCR methods have some disadvantages such as cumbersome, labor intensive, slow or have low test throughput or turn around times (Stone and Mahnoy, 2014). Loop-mediated isothermal amplification (LAMP) is a novel isothermal nucleic acid amplification method which is commonly used for the amplification of DNAs and RNAs, with great sensitivity and high specificity (Notomi et al., 2000; Enosawa et al., 2003), which has been developed into commercially available detection kits for a variety of pathogens such as bacteria and viruses (Mori and Notomi, 2009). LAMP technique has the potential to revolutionize molecular biology due to DNA amplification under isothermal conditions in this method (Zhang et al., 2014). The goal of this manuscript is to review molecular detection and PCR as an important tool in biological research and detection of toxins, pathogens and infectious organisms.

Chapter 2

Molecular Detection

Nucleic acid based amplification approaches such as polymerase chain reaction (PCR), nucleic acid sequence-based amplification (NASBA), transcription mediated amplification (TMA), strand displacement amplification (SDA), loop-mediated isothermal amplification (LAMP), rolling circle amplification (RCA), helicase dependent amplification (HAD), and multiplex ligation-dependent probe amplification (MLPA) have been used for the detection of viruses. Isothermal amplification methods can achieve highly sensitive and specific nucleic acid detection, and it has overcome the need of sophisticated thermal equipment and elongated thermal cycling protocols (Deng et al., 2017, Yang et al., 2019). Different isothermal amplification methods are shown in Table 1.

Immunoassays such as Enzyme-linked immune-sorbent assay (ELISA) rely on the use of antibodies, conjugates, and enzymes which are costly and require lengthy incubation times and special conditions for their storage (Gan and Patel, 2013; Rizvi et al., 2020). With the increasing demand for multiplexed molecular detection, encoded particles have evolved from pattern encoding to signal-intensity encoding, and also from signal-molecule encapsulation to signal-molecule tagging (Li and Luo, 2006). The demand for remote molecular detection has been rising in recent years (Liu et al., 2020). Amagliani et al., (2012) found that molecular detection has the potential to screen large numbers of environmental samples, and could be proposed as part of a self-monitoring plant for recreational facilities, improving surveillance and early warning systems. Molecular detection of resistance to antituberculosis drugs is a significantly faster approach that has reduced turnaround time for detecting drug resistance (Bwanga et al., 2009). Molecular testing of drug resistance is based on the detection of mutations altering genes or the expression of genes associated with the development of drug resistance (Brossier et al., 2017). Targeted molecular MRI combines the advantages of high spatial resolution and contrast without the need for ionizing radiation making it an attractive imaging technique to study molecular processes (Gilchrist et al., 2020). The storage temperature, storage duration and the type of swab could be critical parameters for successful isolation or molecular detection (Ball et al., 2020). Li et al., (2020) concluded that based on the catalytic amplifying strategy and the TMB diimine molecular probes, ultratrace Fe^{3+} could be also detected by SERS and fluorescence methods. The small subunit ribosomal RNA (18S rRNA) gene has been widely used for species identification, phylogenetic and genotype studies in *Theileria equi* and *Babesia caballi* (Hall et al., 2013; Qablan et al., 2013; Seo et al., 2013; Veronesi et al., 2014; Braga et al., 2017; Peckle et al., 2018; Vieira et al., 2018). Wang et al., (2019) reported that the molecular epidemiological and genetic diversity results provide important epidemiological data for control equine piroplasmosis caused by *T. equi* and *B. caballi* in China. Molecular techniques can be utilized to more definitively screen germ-free (GF) and selectively colonized animals for bacterial contamination when gram stain and/or culture results are un-interpretable or inconsistent (Packey et al., 2013). Molecular beacon techniques are attractive for biosensing and bioassays for nucleic acids, showing advantages in sensitivity, simplicity and rapidity (Wang et al., 2019). Akashi et al., (2019) reported a high performance of Liat for the rapid molecular identification of the influenza virus. Zhang et al., (2019) utilized molecular beacon-based fluorescence in situ hybridization (MB-FISh) for rapid and direct detection of *Staphylococcus aureus* in positive blood cultures. Laboratory approaches for the detection of quinolone resistance are based on phenotypic methods and molecular methods (Abou El-Khier and El-Sayed Zaki, 2020). Molecular techniques used for recognition of quinolone resistance consist of the use of various techniques such as polymerase chain reaction fragment length polymorphism (Nakano et al., 2013), multiplex real-time PCR (Kim et al., 2012), single-stranded conformation polymorphism (SSCP) (Deborah et al., 2002), nucleotide-sequencing analysis and multiplex allele-specific polymerase chain reaction (MAS-PCR) (Onseedaeng and Ratthawongjirakul, 2016). Specific oligonucleotide primers can be designed and used for molecular detection of bacterial contaminants in both tissue cultures of *B. magnifica* ssp. *acutisepalia*, and in other plants (Tsoktouridis et al., 2014). Mousavi et al., (2017) reported that molecular detection can be used as a simple diagnostic kit in clinical laboratories for identification of *Vibrio cholera*. Nelson et al., (2019) concluded that rapid genomic diagnostics in a clinical setting is a rapid and cost-effective tool to track antibiotic resistance in both pathogens and strains.

Table 1. Different isothermal amplification methods

Methods	Samples	References
The signal amplification assays	Rapid isothermal nucleic acid detection assays (RIDA)	Gao et al., (2008)
	Catalyzed hairpin assembly (CHA)	Li et al., (2011) Yin et al., (2008)
	Signal mediated amplification of RNA technology (SMART)	Tyagi and Kramer (1996) Tyagi and Bratu (1998) Wharam et al., (2001) Hall et al., (2002)
The probe amplification assays	Invader assays	Kwiatkowski et al., (1999) Allawai et al., (2004) Duffy et al., (2008)
The target amplification assays	Nucleic acid sequence-based amplification (NASBA)	Bremer et al., (2000) Polstra et al., (2002) Guichon et al., (2004)
	Helicase-dependent amplification (HAD)	An et al., (2005) Gill et al., (2006) Gill et al., (2007)
	Isothermal multiple displacement amplification (IMDA)	Lasken and Egholm (2003) Luthra and Medeiros (2004)
	Loop-mediated isothermal amplification (LAMP)	Enosawa et al., (2003) Parida et al., (2004)
	Single primer isothermal amplification (SPIA)	Kurn et al., (2005) Singh et al., (2005)
	Strand displacement amplification (SDA)	Little et al., (1999)
	Rolling circle amplification (RCA)	Dean et al., (2001) Demidov (2002) Cho et al., (2005)

Smoothing spline clustering (SSC) method was a suggested method to estimate the highly variable sites for the evolution study of infectious bronchitis virus (IBV). Surface-enhanced Raman scattering (SERS) has been a powerful and attractive spectroscopic technique for molecular detection due to its label-free identification of chemicals from their specific Raman spectra and significant Raman signal enhancement of target molecules adsorbed onto novel plasmonic metal nanostructures (Cao et al., 2002; Anker et al., 2008; Reokrungruang et al., 2019; Haldavnekar et al., 2020); it also shows many benefits such as low cost, flexibility, portability and biodegradability (Li et al., 2013; Yetisen et al., 2013; Zhang et al., 2014; Kim et al., 2018), and the developed paper-based SERS sensor is expected to be applicable as a label-free sensor for a variety of chemical and biological molecules (Linh et al., 2019). Molecular detection of *Mycobacterium leprae* in clinical and environmental samples has been reported using a variety of target sequences using both conventional and real time-PCR formats (Tatipally et al., 2018). Ferreira et al., (2020), after molecular detection of infection with *Mycobacterium leprae* in six Brazilian banded armadillos (*Euphractus sexcinctus*), reported that in common with *Dasypus novemcinctus*, six banded armadillos represent a potential reservoir of *M. leprae* and as such, their role in a possible zoonotic cycle of leprosy within Brazil warrants further investigation. Molecularly imprinted polymer-based sensors detection possesses unique properties which offer significant advantages for food safety hazard factors detection (FSHFs) (Cao et al., 2019), and it can also recognize both small molecules and various macromolecular targets, including proteins, viruses, and also microorganisms.

Chapter 3

Molecular Detection and Epidemic Diseases

Epidemic disease outbreaks are a major threat to human society, and suppressing and preventing epidemic spreading is of critical importance to the well being of the human society (Yang et al., 2019). Re-emerging or novel infectious diseases usually first occur in a certain population or geographic area, and then they can swiftly disperse locally or globally (Christaki, 2015). Vector-borne viruses are divided into four groups on the basis of genome characteristics, namely, single-stranded negative sense RNA, single-stranded positive sense RNA, double-stranded RNA and DNA (Cholleti et al., 2018). Early detection is essential for disease control mitigation, as timely reactions are generally more successful and less detrimental for the host population (Cunniffe et al., 2016; Bourhis et al., 2019). Molecular assays consist of three main steps: specimen processing (DNA or RNA extraction); nucleic acid amplification; and detection of amplified product (Jaton-Ogay and Bille, 2008). Molecular diagnostics of infectious diseases are based on nucleic acid assay methods. Nucleic acid testing techniques are shown in Table 2.

Nucleic acid amplification strategies and advances in amplicon detection methodologies have been the key factors in the progress of molecular microbiology (Mangal et al., 2016). Detection and diagnosis of prion diseases, include some human diseases, is contingent upon developing assays, which exploit properties uniquely possessed by this misfolded protein complex, rather than targeting an agent-specific nucleic acid (Lehto et al., 2006). Kost (2018) reported that the key important for highly infectious diseases is lack of community rapid response and resilience which should be enhanced by molecular diagnostics directly at critical points of need. Nucleotide sequencing and laboratory automation have aided the introduction of many methods and provided accurate and portable data (Diggle and Clarke, 2006). Shi and Kramer (2003) found that surveillance techniques employing nucleic acid-based assays have played an essential role in monitoring the spread of West Nile virus. The immune-polymerase chain reaction (IPCR) method has the potential to become the most analytically sensitive method available for the detection of target proteins of infectious diseases (Barletta and Bartolome, 2007).

Table 2. Nucleic acid testing techniques

Main categories	Sub-categories	Methods	Characteristics	Reference
Amplified nucleic acid techniques	Target amplification	1. PCR 2. Transcription-based methods (TBM) 3. Strand displacement amplification-LAMP (SDA)	a. PCR is the most common target amplification method to detect cultures and uncultured bacteria. b. PCR amplification based techniques which have been designed for bacterial detections and identifications are competitive PCR, most probable number PCR (MPN-PCR), co-operational PCR, BIO-PCR, nested-PCR and real-time PCR. c. Real-time PCR is the most useful and fast method with lower contamination risk and higher sensitivity. d. Unlike PCR, transcription based methods and strand displacement amplification are isothermal techniques that do not require a thermal cycler. e. The most important benefits of amplification methods are the requirement for low target copy number within a direct specimen.	Cobo (2012) Schmitt and Barroca (2012)
	Signal amplification	1. Branched DNA 2. Hybrid capture	a. In the last two decades, hybrid capture has become a popular technique applicable to gynecological cytology specimens. b. The method entails the reaction between DNA-RNA hybrids and anti-hybrid antibodies with a luminometer measuring the light emitted.	Muldrew (2009) Cobo (2012)
	Probe amplification techniques	1. Ligase chain reaction 2. Cycling probe technology 3. Clvease-invading technology		

Main categories	Sub-categories	Methods	Characteristics	Reference
Microarrays		1. DNA microarrays 2. Multiplex microsphere-based array	a. These techniques provide rapid diagnoses with a decreased contamination risk, low cost, high sensitivity and specificity and rapid kinetics through the use of a closed-tube systems.	Fenollar and Raoult (2004) Weile and Knabbe (2009) Cobo (2012) Schmitt and Barroca (2012)
Non-amplified nucleic acid techniques	DNA labeled probes		a. These techniques are safe, sensitive, simple and specific in detecting and identifying the microorganisms directly from the clinical specimen such as a smear.	Barken et al., (2007)
	RNA labeled probes			

Decousser et al., (2017) showed that given the availability of fully automated wet and dry whole genome sequencing solutions, microbiologists should focus on inexpensive biochemical tests for cultured isolated or monomicrobial clinical specimen. Molecular-based methods offer a great chance to improve detection of drug-resistant pathogens, but it is important to have a profound understanding of drug resistance mechanisms and circulating different strains (Engstrom, 2016). Molecular methods have considerable advantages for the programmatic management of drug resistance (Ramachandran and Muniyandi, 2018). Taha (2002) concluded that molecular approaches of typing allow a reliable tracking of meningococcal strains and a powerful epidemiological analysis. Lemieux et al., (2012) reported that the near instrument-free, rapid and simple characteristics of the IsoAmp HSV assay make it potentially suitable for point-of care testing. The duplex real-time PCR assay was introduced as a sensitive, specific and reproducible method for differentiating of porcine epidemic diarrhea virus (PEDV) (Zheng et al., 2020). Real-time analysis, high sensitivity, miniaturization, rapid detection time and low-cost biosensor technologies are appropriate for the diagnosis of epidemic diseases in animals (Du and Zhou, 2018).

The ARIES influenza A/B/RSV assay is a specific and rapid molecular assay because its performance in clinical samples is comparable to laboratory-developed automated real-time RT-PCR assays (LDA) and better than those of the established rapid assays (Voermans et al., 2016). Lalle et al., (2010) confirmed that the novel nucleoprotein reverse-transcription-PCR showed higher sensitivity for A/H1N1pdm than a commercial test for influenza A. Vries et al., (2013) suggested RT-PCR assays as a powerful tool for enhanced influenza virus surveillance. Budiarto et al., (2019) reported that three platforms of molecular detection systems have been employed in finding the evidence of HER2^{I655V} SNP in breast carcinogenesis where PCR-RFLP and TaqMan Assay have become molecular assays which are widely used for this purpose. NAT tests can detect the viruses sooner than serologic tests, and this assay has a wide variability to accurately provide results on cadaveric specimens (Ribeiro et al., 2019). Ibrahim et al., (2020) found that the multiplex nested PCR had identified Occult HBV infection (OBI) with a high rate supporting the efficiency of using molecular techniques in detecting of hepatitis B virus (HBV) which will lead to an appropriate diagnosis and minimizing the risk to be infected by HBV.

Chapter 4

Molecular Detection of COVID-19

Viral RNA shedding of SARS-CoV-2 occurred in multiple tissues including the respiratory system, blood and intestine, and variable levels of specific anti-SARS-CoV-2 antibody may be associated with disease severity (Li et al., 2020). Understanding the molecular mechanisms of how SARS-CoV-2 interacts with host cells and stimulates the immune response is an important strategy for development and progress of specific COVID-19 therapies and vaccines (Alnefaie and Albogami, 2020). RT-PCR and serology tests have been used for diagnosis of COVID-19, and biosensor-based methods are under development for SARS-CoV-2 and many challenges still exist in diagnostic methods, including the accuracy (Teklemariam et al., 2020). Ishige et al., (2020) a developed multiplex rRT-PCR which will enable reducing agent use and cost and handling time for SARS-CoV-2 RNA detection. Colombian SARS-CoV-2 sequences displayed genetic variability in some target regions used for COVID-19 diagnosis, and genomic data of circulating SARS-CoV-2 allow the refinement of molecular protocols for COVID-19 diagnosis (Alvarez-Diaz et al., 2020). Liotti et al., (2020) suggested that the lower analytical sensitivity of the BioFire COVID-19 test might have caused false-negative results in studies, and relying on fully automated FilmArray platforms, BioFire COVID-19 test provides results in approximately 45 minutes from N/OP sample collection. Sakanashi et al., (2020) proposed that saliva can potentially serve as an alternative to nasopharyngeal swabs as a specimen for SARS-CoV-2 rRT-PCR. Multiple molecular assays such as Altona, the CDC assay and GenMark were developed for the detection of SARS-CoV-2 (Uhteg et al., 2020).

Mostafa et al., (2020) compared the analytical sensitivities of seven SARS-CoV-2 molecular assays and found that the Abbott, the Roche, and the Xpert Xpress assays appear more sensitive. Rodel et al., (2020) reported that variplex RT-LAMP may serve as a rapid test to be combined with an RT-PCR assay to increase the diagnostic accuracy in patients with suspected COVID-19 infection. Afzal et al., (2020) reported that small-footprint rapid test equipment for cost-effective point-of-care diagnosis of COVID-19 are being developed as Abbott's famous ID NOW™ Instrument and ID NOW™

COVID-19 Test Kit and Lumex Instruments' Microchip RT-PCR COVID-19 Detection System.

Chapter 5

Rapid Detection

The novel PCR-based method has high sensitivity and specificity, but several molecular tests which employ non-PCR-based methods are developed for rapid detection of RNA such as isothermal nucleic acid amplification (loop mediated isothermal amplification (LAMP), and nucleic acid sequence-based amplification) (Shen et al., 2020). The real-time polymerase chain reaction detection results corresponded closely to visual assessments of diseases severity (Zhao et al., 2012). The rapid internally-controlled PCR assay is recommended for *Bordetella pertussis* and *Bordetella parapertussis* (Slinger et al., 2011). It has been reported that rapid, selective and sensitive detection of nucleic acids and proteins are important for the identification or pathogens of food safety importance providing inspecting evidence, and for the identification of known genotypes using hybrid biological/inorganic devices (Fauci, 2002, Patolsky et al., 2004; Van den heuvel and dekker, 2007). Wang et al., (2020) also concluded that rapid detection of food-borne pathogens is crucial to prevent the outbreaks of food-borne illnesses (Du et al., 2019; Wang et al., 2020). The most important methods which can be used to detect the pathogens are biochemical assays, immunological assays, and polymerase chain reaction (PCR)-based testing of bacterial nucleic acids (Zhang et al., 2013).

The resazurin microplate method can be used as a reliable, easy, cheap and rapid method for early detection of vancomycin-resistant enterococci (VRE) which are a serious challenge for physicians because of the limited treatment options for infections (Coban et al., 2005). Cockerill (2003) reported that nucleic acid-based testing methods, compared with conventional culture-based methods, have the potential to provide much more rapid detection of pathogens and determination of antimicrobial resistance for the infections caused by methicillin-resistant *Staphylococcus aureus* (MRSA), VRE, and extended spectrum beta-lactamase (ESBL) producing gram-negative bacilli. Taguri et al., (2011) found that a rapid detection method can be used for *Legionella* control at bathing facilities. Rapid detection for psychotrophic microorganisms is also important for ensuring food safety and quality for cold storage foods (Wei et al., 2019). A sol-gel molecularly imprinted polymer (MIP) film and a simple quartz crystal microbalance (QCM) sensor and HPLC-MS method may indicate the developed method which can accurately detect patulin in practical food samples (Fang et al., 2016). Sun et al., (2017) after molecular detection of Torque teno canis virus (TTCaV) in domestic dogs suggested that TTCaV has a large genetic diversity and showed that TTCaV and canine parvovirus (CPV) co-infection exists in China. The most important bacteria detection methods are colorimetric detection (Srisaart et al., 2018; Alamer et al., 2018), fluorescence detection (Duan et al., 2015; Giovaninni et al., 2018), and electrochemical detection (Liu et al., 2016; Liu et al., 2017). Effective rapid detection methods also necessary to determine chemical hazards mainly because of their high toxicity (Arvanitoyannis et al., 2014; Khaled et al., 2015; Xing et al., 2019). It has been used for detection of mercury and iodine (Wang et al., 2015). Fluorescence polarization immunoassay (FPIA) is a rapid, sensitive, specific and simple method for the quantitative detection of Bisphenol A in environmental water samples (Wu et al., 2012). Das et al., (2020) reported an aptamer-NanoZyme-based assay for possible applications to detect *Escherichia coli* contamination in the juice product. Hiremath et al., (2020) found that a novel carbon dots-MnO_2 assembly based fluorescent probe is an alternative to existing detection tools for on-site detection and quantification of hydrazine.

The technique of rtPCR may allow rapid detection and quantification of the pathogen DNA at the pictogram level in soils and in plants, facilitating the screening of the pathogen in diverse areas (Mirmajlessi et al., 2016). Rapid real-time PCR diagnosis can result in appropriate control measures and eradication procedures more quickly and accurately than traditional methods of pathogen isolation (Schaad and Frederick, 2002). A sensitive immunochromatographic assay (ICA) using a colloidal gold-antibody probe was applied for the rapid detection of fumonisin B_1 (FB_1) in corn samples (Wang et al., 2016). Rapid detection on the basis of microscopic observations and morphological identification is recommended for *Esteya vermicola*, which is an endoparasitic fungus of the pinewood nematode (Wei et al., 2014). A surface-enhanced Raman scattering (SERS) approach based on silver-coated gold nanoparticles was applied as a rapid detection method of multiple organophosphorus pesticides such as triazophos and methyl-parathion in peach fruit (Yaseen et al., 2019).

Li et al., (2009) introduced a rapid detection strip as a sensitive, specific, and easy-to-use method for the quantitative, semi-quantitative or qualitative detection of sulfamethazine residues in swine urine. Geng et al., (2019) recommended recombinase polymerase amplification (RPA) for the detection of *Campylobacter jejuni*, which is the most frequently reported bacterial food-borne pathogen in human gastrointestinal infections (Kaakoush et al., 2015). Culture-independent methods have been developed for rapid detection of *Staphylococcus aureus*, including ELISA (Nouri et al., 2018), PCR (Zeng et al., 2016), real-time multiplex PCR (Alhaj et al., 2009), and loop-mediated isothermal amplification (LAMP) (Sheet et al., 2016). Molecular and metabolic strategies of heat-resistant fungus detection and identification are complementary and can be used to measure postharvest quality of fruit and their products (Pertile et al., 2020). Rapid detection and identification of heat-resistant fungus belonging to genera Byssochlamys and Hamigera (Nakayama et al., 2010), Byssochlamys (Hosoya et al., 2012), Neosartorya (Yaguchi et al., 2012), and Talaromyces (Panek and Frac, 2018) were used. Recombinase polymerase amplification coupled with lateral flow dipstick (RPA-LED) assay can be used as a rapid and sensitive method to monitor *Karlodinium veneficum* (Fu et al., 2019). RPA-LFD assay was already used for diagnostic tests of toxins in food samples (Shiu et al., 2019), infective parasites (Nair et al., 2015; Rosser et al., 2015), pathogenic bacteria (Ma et al., 2017), and viruses (Tu et al., 2017). Several rapid detection methods have been developed to monitor the presence of microorganisms such as ATP bioluminescence (Fratamico et al., 2011; Law et al., 2015), and catalase activity-based method (Sippy et al., 2003) to detect the mold, bacteria, and pathogens in food products (Valat et al., 2003). Ziyaina et al., (2020) proposed rapid microbial investigation methods that may replace conventional product quality testing techniques in the dairy industry. Biosensor-based detection methods are a potential alternative to conventional culture-dependent enumeration techniques and various portable sensors have been developed to analyze the microbial activity in foods (Jayan et al., 2020).

Chapter 6

Rapid Detection of COVID-19

The rapid diagnosis of COVID-19 patients is essential to reduce the disease spread (Mak et al., 2020). A modified CDC-based laboratory developed test is able to detect SARS-CoV-2 accurately with similar sensitivity across all sample types tested (Perchetti et al., 2020). Detection of SARS-CoV-2 within 3.5 h (sample-to-answer-time) by random access real time PCR and differentiation of SARS-CoV-2 with a PCR for the EdRp Gene had been adopted (Cordes and Heim, 2020). Zhen and Berry (2020) demonstrated that the Northwell Health Laboratories laboratory developed test (NWHL LDT) multiplex assay performs as well as the modified CDC assay, and it is more efficient and cost effective for epidemiological surveillance and clinical management of SARS-CoV-2. A simple method to detect SARS-CoV-2 from specimens is inactivating samples by heating and precipitating with a PEG/NaCl solution before rRT-PCR assay for Orflab, N and S genes, and this new method could be compared with an automated protocol of nucleic acid extraction (Ulloa et al., 2020). Barza et al., (2020) reported that a simple heat-RNA release method is a reasonable alternative for the majority of COVID-19 positive patients which can help overcome the cost and availability issues of RNA extraction reagents. Wu et al., (2020) observed that the real-time RT-RAA assay may be a valuable tool for detecting SARS-CoV-2. Rahimi et al., (2020) considered PCR-approaches (RT-PCR) as the most reliable options, and CRISPR/Cas-based approaches as the most sensitive and less costly molecular techniques for detection of SARS-CoV-2.

CRISPR-based novel techniques, when merged with isothermal and allied technologies, promise to provide sensitive and rapid detection of SARS-CoV-2 nucleic acids; they can also open a future avenue for development of low-cost, rapid, sensitive, accurate and suitable point of care diagnostics (Javalkote et al., 2020). Bordi et al., (2020) concluded that a newly designed real-time RT-PCR (Simplexa^{TM} COVID-19 Direct assay) is promising for laboratory diagnosis, enabling highspeed detection in just over hours which allows prompt decision making regarding isolation of infected patients. Two quantitative automated immunoassays (Maglumi^{TM} 2019-n-CoV IgC and IgM and Euroimmune Anti-SARS-CoV-2 IgG and IgA assays) and their lateral flow rapid tests were performed. Euroimmune ELISA IgG/IgA tests show higher overall sensitivity than Maglumi CLIA IgG/IgM tests. Maglumi CLIA IgM test shows 100% specificity, and lateral flow tests show similar overall performance as Euroimmun ELISA IgG/IgA and Maglumi CLIA IgG/IgM test (Montesinos et al., 2020). Xing et al., (2020) successfully developed a high-throughput nucleic acid isothermal amplification system which was capable of detecting 19 common respiratory viruses, including SARS-CoV-2, within 90 min; they have reported that RTisochip^{TM}-W system can be utilized as a powerful nucleic acid testing tool in the diagnosis and screening of SARS-CoV-2, especially when the precise cause of pneumonia is urgently demanded. Porte et al., (2020) concluded that rapid antigen detection has the potential to become an important tool for the early diagnosis of SARS-CoV-2, particularly in situations with limited access to molecular methods, and the rapid antigen detection test evaluated has a high diagnostic sensitivity and specificity in respiratory samples obtained from patients who mainly presented during the first week of COVID-19. RT-PCR protocol was suitable for all respiratory materials, and high SARS-CoV-2 detection rate by direct RT-qPCR of 95.8% for Ct values <35 was reported (Lubke et al., 2020). A portable microfluidic ELISA technology for rapid (15 min), quantitative, and sensitive detection of anti-SARS-CoV-2 S1 IgG in human serum with only 8 μL sample volume was recommended, because knowing the concentration of SARS-CoV-2 S1-specific IgG is crucial in selecting appropriate convalescent serum donors (Tan et al., 2020). Michel et al., (2020) reported that COVID-quick-DET might be best suited for countries with general shortage or temporary acute scarcity of resources and equipment, which is rapid, reliable, and cost-effective and could bypass or temporally bridge shortage of resources. Ali et al., (2020) reported that RT-LAMP coupled with CRISPR-Cas12 (iSCAN) provides a sensitive and specific virus detection platform, and iSCAN sensitivity and specificity are comparable with RT-qPCR and it is a 1 h detection module which can help in testing in low resource areas and developed as a one-pot assay. Different nucleic acid amplification tests of COVID-19 are shown in Table 3.

Table 3. Different nucleic acid amplification tests of COVID-19

Methods	Key points	Reference
Reverse transcription polymerase chain reaction (RT-PCR)	a. It was the first method developed for COVID-19 which has been adopted by WHO in different countries. b. Analytical accuracy of COVID-19 RT-PCR relies primarily on the primer deign. Identifying unique gene sequences is important to eliminate cross-reactivity. c. Viral targets RNAse P (RP) are used for internal positive control. d. RT-PCR tests are usually performed in centralized laboratories due to the requirement of dedicated equipment and stringent contamination control, which offer both high accuracy and throughput	Corman et al., (2020) Jung et al., (2020) Sohrabi et al., (2020) Xia et al., (2020)
Digital PCR based COVID-19 detection	a. Digital PCR enables the absolute quantification of target nucleic acids, and partitions samples into large numbers of small reaction volumes, ensuring that each partition contains a few or no= target sequences per Poisson's statistics. b. Droplet Digital PCR (ddPCR) is the most widely used method with commercial systems available. c. ddPCR reported decrease in viral loads of specimens collected from different locations of the same patient.	Dong et al., (2020) Lu et al., (2020)
Loop-mediated isothermal amplification (LAMP)	a. LAMP uses 4 or 6 primers, targeting 6-8 regions in the genome, and Bsm DNA polymerase. b. Primer sets targeting regions of COVID-19 ORF1a and N genes.	Park et al., (2020) Yu et al., (2020) Zhu et al., (2020)
Nicking endonuclease amplification reaction (NEAR)	a. NEAR uses both strand-displacement DNA polymerase and nicking endonuclease enzymes to exponentially amplify short oligonucleotides.	Menova et al., (2013) Nie et al., (2014)
Recombinase polymerase amplification (RPA)	a. RPA borrows its concept from homologous DNA recombination to amplify double-stranded DNA. b. For COVID-19, RPA primers have been designed targeting regions of N gene.	Xia and Chen (2020)
Clustered regularly interspaced short palindromic repeats (CRISPR)	a. CRISPR systems offer new ways to amplify analytical signal with the precision down to single-nucleotide variants. b. Cas12a and Cas13-based COVID-19 test designed for COVID-19 detection.	Aman et al., (2020) Broughton et al., (2020) Metsky et al., (2020)

Chapter 7

PCR

PCR technology has emerged as a basic tool in biological research and in the detection of infectious organisms, and has the potential to provide information on a number of toxins and virulence factors as well as allow species identification of pathogens (Singh, 2003). With the invention of polymerase chain reaction (PCR) in the 1980s, it became possible to replicate nucleic acids, and PCR technology depends on numerous cycles of heating and cooling (Beal et al., 2016). Quantitative real-time PCR tests have been extensively developed in clinical microbiology laboratories for routine diagnosis of infectious diseases, especially bacterial diseases (Maurin, 2012). PCR-based method has become a routine and reliable technique for detecting coronaviruses (Balboni et al., 2012; Uhlenhaut et al., 2012). The real-time RT-PCR assay is a predominant method to be applied for the detection of all kinds of coronaviruses (Corman et al., 2012; Lu et al., 2014; Corman et al., 2020). PCR involves amplification of a specific gene or genes, and the amplified product is then detected qualitatively or quantitatively (Tan et al., 2020). Compared to the protein-based method, PCR is less compromised by conditions associated with food processing, and it is also simple, rapid, specific and sensitive (Lockley and Bardsley, 2000). Real-time quantitative PCR (qPCR) is even more sensitive (Navarro et al., 2015). The reliability and sensitivity of PCR assays depend on DNA quality (Cseke et al., 2011; Talley and Cseke, 2011).

PCR is also a powerful technique that revolutionized molecular biology by offering applications in the diagnosis of microbial infections and genetic diseases, as well as in detection of pathogens in food (Calvo et al., 2001). Real-time PCR seems as sensitive but less prone to contamination as amplification and detection occurs, and it is easy to perform, rapid and easy to automate, but nested PCR is too prone to contamination (Jaton-Ogay and Bille, 2008). Testing for several viruses requires a series of monoplex PCRs, which can be both expensive and time-consuming, while the use of multiplex assays may significantly reduce the hands-on time and cost (Mansuy et al., 2012). The most important techniques for food-borne pathogen detection are DNA hybridization or gene probe assays consisting of detection of DNA or

RNA targets using complementary labeled nucleic acid probes, DNA microarray (also named DNA chip or biochip), nucleic acid sequence based amplification (NASBA), randomly amplified polymorphic DNA (RAPD) which is another PCR based technique, and amplified fragment length polymorphism (AFLP) which is mainly used for molecular typing and detecting restriction fragments of the genome using PCR (Boughattas and Salehi, 2014). Although PCR as a molecular method is specific and sensitive, the technique is time-intensive, while the real-time PCR method can be more specific but involves complex processing steps and requires prior sequence data of the specific target gene (Smith and Osborn, 2009).

Multiplex PCR (M-PCR) is the simultaneous detection of more than one target sequence. It has a potential to produce considerable savings of time and effort within the laboratory without compromising test utility (Kalvatchev et al., 2004). M-PCR has been shown to be a valuable method for identification of bacteria, fungi, viruses and parasites (Kalvatchev et al., 2004). Multiplex PCR assays are basic tools for the simultaneous detection of toxins, virulence factors and pathogens in clinical and environmental specimens (Singh, 2003; Mohapatra et al., 2011). A newly developed semi-nested PCR (snPCR) method has been introduced for detection of scale drop disease virus (SDDV) (Charoenwai et al., 2019). Real-time PCR methodology can be employed for the rapid detection of the four most prevalent hand, foot and mouth disease (HFMD)-associated enteroviruses (Evs), for epidemiologic surveillance of circulating EV genotypes and for assessing treatment responses and vaccine studies (Wang et al., 2018b). The real-time PCR assay can facilitate disease management by providing early and accurate diagnosis of the bleeding canker disease of pear (Tian et al., 2020). The nest-PCR is a novel, useful and convenient method with high sensitivity and specificity (Huang et al., 2019). There are two types of fluorogenic PCR-based detection methods: one of the assays utilizes the 5′ nuclease activity of *Taq* DNA polymerase to hydrolyse an internal fluorogenic probe for monitoring amplification of DNA target (Hoofar et al., 2000; Rodriguez-Lazaro et al., 2003), while the other iQ-Check system utilized a fluorogenic probe which has flanking GC-rich arm sequences complementary to one another (Chen et al., 2000; Liming and Bhagwat, 2004), and in both types of real-time PCR probes, a fluorescent moiety is conjugated to one end of the sequence, and a quencher moiety is attached to the other end of the sequence (Patel et al., 2006). Nucleic acid amplification tests (NAATs), such as polymerase chain reaction (PCR) and real-time quantitative PCR (qPCR), have been widely applied to detect food-borne

Salmonella due to the sensitivity and rapid detection capabilities of these assays (Chiu et al., 2005; Bansal et al., 2006; Hein et al., 2006; McGuinness et al., 2009; Almeida et al., 2013). Many qPCR assays have been published which provide useful information for the infectious bursal disease virus (IBDV) (Kong et al., 2009; Ghorashi et al., 2011; Jayasundara et al., 2017; Kurukulasuriya et al., 2017; Tomas et al., 2017) and the chicken anemia virus (CAV) (Davidson et al., 2013; Varela et al., 2014; Olszewska-Tomczyk et al., 2016) diagnosis and characterization. qPCR techniques are excellent alternatives because they are fast, sensitive, and adaptable to a multiplex format for highly specific target detection of more than one viral genome in a single reaction (Tomas et al., 2012; Marandino et al., 2016). The qPCR assays can be used in simplex and duplex formats for detection and quantification of large number of samples with reliable sensitivity and specificity (Techera et al., 2019).

The direct TaqMan qPCR assay possesses high specificity, sensitivity and reproducibility, indicating that it can be used as a powerful tool for detection and quantification of various carnivore amdoparvoviruses in epidemiological and pathogenesis studies (Wu et al., 2019). It has been reported that the sensitivity and specificity of conventional PCR is lower than qPCR (Farid and Rupasinghe, 2017). Tayebeh et al., (2017) reported on polymerase chain reaction-enzyme linked immunosorbent assay (PCR-ELISA) as a simple manner for detection of microorganism such as bacteria, viruses, fungi, and others based on nucleic acid sequence. Multiplex PCR has been found effective for simultaneously detecting *Salmonella* and other pathogens in foods, especially with real-time PCR (Levin, 2009). Linton et al., (1997) used PCR to identify and differentiate between *Campylobacter jejuni* and *C. coli* in diarrheic samples. Fratamico et al., (2000) used multiplex PCR to detect *E. coli* O157:H7 in foods and in bovine feces using targets specific for the H serogroup and specific genes associated with O157 specific virulence factors. DNA hybridization techniques have been used in the detection and identification of food-borne pathogens (Hill et al., 1998), mainly with the extensive use of polymerase chain reaction (PCR) (Kim et al., 2007). The immunomagnetic separation (IMS) PCR detection method was considered quite sensitive, rapid and reliable and could be applied to the detection of *Cronobacter* in foods (Tram et al., 2012; Chen et al., 2017). De Boer et al., (2010) reported that results of multiple real-time PCR assays may provide valuable information for patient management and minimizing the spread of the hypervirulent epidemic 027/NAP1 strain. BNA Real-time PCR Mutation Detection Kit Extended RAS (BNA Real-time PCR) has been considered as a valuable tool for predicting the efficacy of early anti-formalin-fixed paraffin-embedded (EGFR) therapy in metastatic colorectal cancer (mCRC) patients (Iida et al., 2019). Reverse transcriptase polymerase chain reaction (RT-PCR) is an important technique which may help effectively control Newcastle disease (Li et al., 2009). It is also a promising tool for molecular epidemiological studies of foot and mouth disease virus (FMDV) (Le et al., 2012; Wernike et al., 2013). Evagreen-based fluorescence quantitative real-time RT-PCR assay is an important method which may benefit the investigation of possible sporadic outbreaks of calicivirus (CV) infections in geese as well as epidemiological and etiological studies of goose-origin CV (GCVs) (Lin et al., 2020).

The first line system for the detection of foot-and-mouth disease virus (FMDV) from the sample materials is real time quantitative RT-PCR (RT-qPCR) (Callahan et al., 2002; Reid et al., 2003). Fontel et al., (2019) found that diagnosis of foot-and-mouth disease (FMD) can be achieved using EDTA-stabilized blood samples in an outbreak situation on the herb basis, but serum is preferred at the single animal level for optimal sensitivity. Multiplex RT-PCR amplification is a useful tool for the detection and characterization of plant viruses (Mumford et al., 2006; Yang et al., 2017). Qian et al., (2018) proposed a duplex and visual method using rapid PCR combined with molecular beacons to specifically detect two kinds of shrimp pathogens in one reaction tube, which may give a possibility to conduct end-point visual duplex detection. The developed rapid polymerase chain reaction (PCR) has a great potential for rapid on-site detection of pork meat and identification meat species (Wu et al., 2020). Rapid PCR have been used to conduct molecular diagnosis of bacteria, virus or genetically modified organisms (Houssin et al., 2016; Qian et al., 2018 a,b,c). The higher sensitivity of PCR method is recommended for diagnosis of anaplasmosis, especially in carrier animals (Jalili et al., 2013). A real-time reverse transcription-polymerase chain reaction (RT-PCR) was used to detect MuV F gene, and characterization was performed by sequencing of the SH gene of mumps virus (MuV) (Brauer et al., 2016). Kuypers (2010) reported the use of RT-PCR assays for the detection of rhinoviruses in clinical specimens which was provided more accurate information about the disease burden and epidemiology of these ubiquitous viruses.

Chapter 8

Loop-Mediated Isothermal Amplification

Loop-mediated isothermal amplification (LAMP), a kind of isothermal deoxyribonucleic acid (DNA) amplification method, is one of the promising approaches for on-site nucleic acid detection because of its high sensitivity, simplicity and high specificity (Notomi et al., 2000). Both DNA and RNA viruses can be detected by LAMP and diagnose various important emerging and re-emerging diseases (Kalvatchev et al., 2010). This technique is a promising alternative to traditional DNA-based diagnostic methods because it can be performed rapidly, it is specific, sensitive and suitable for field diagnostics (Mori and Notomi, 2009; Yang et al., 2010). It is also a promising approach for the rapid and sensitive detection of pathogens, which allows nucleic acid amplification under isothermal conditions (Shang et al., 2020). Kundapur and Nema (2016) reported the implementation of LAMP assay in the field of molecular diagnosis of cancer, identification of genetically modified organisms, detection of food adulteration, eutrophication, food allergens, pesticides, identification of medicinal plants, drug resistance, and DNA methylation studies. This novel nucleic acid amplification method developed by the Eiken Chemical Co., Ltd. (Japan) in 2000 (Cao et al., 2016) can be used in the identification of animal embryo sex, genetically modified foods and various pathogenic organisms (Horisaka et al., 2004; Ohtsuka et al., 2005; Zhao et al., 2010; Wang et al., 2012; Sheu et al., 2018; Girish et al., 2020). LAMP assays have been successfully used for pathogens (Zhao et al., 2011; Kurosaki et al., 2017). The LAMP reaction can be divided into two stages, namely, initial reaction and cyclic reaction, which is driven by four primers, including forward internal primer (FIP), reverse internal primer (BIP), forward outer primer (F3), and reverse outer primer (B3) (Qin et al., 2019). The reaction stages of LAMP are shown in Table 4. Table 5 shows a comparison between PCR and LAMP based methods of viral RNA detection.

Table 4. The reaction stages of LAMP (Notomi et al., 2000, 2015)

1.	In the initial reaction stage, FIP firstly binds complementarily with DNA template.
2.	Extends by polymerization of DNA polymerase with strand displacement activity.
3.	F3 is bound to the DNA template and extends, and the resultant strand will displace the strand of FIP extension at the same time.
4.	The free single-stranded DNA can form a loop structure by complementary sequences within the strand.
5.	Finally, using this single-stranded DNA as the template for the combination and extension of BIP and B3, a new DNA single strand with FIP and BIP is synthesized with DNA polymerase.
6.	The resultant single strand can form a dumbbell-like structure due to the complementary sequence of its two ends.
7.	Then, it enters the stage of cyclic reaction of LAMP and in this stage, a mixture of DNA fragments of polycyclic cauliflower structures with variable sizes are finally produced through intrachain self-cyclization, the incessant binding of primers FIP and BIP, and the strand displacement reaction.

Table 5. Comparison between PCR and LAMP based method of viral RNA detection (Nguyen et al., 2020; Kashir and Yaqinuddin, 2020)

PCR	LAMP
Bulky and cumbersome	Smaller, simpler, portable
Specialised thermal cyclers required	Only a heat block is required
4-8 h until result	1 h until result
Requires skilled technicians	Requires no specific skill
Requires an additional reverse transcription step	Can be performed directly on RNA
Unstable reaction prone to inhibitors requiring purification steps	Stable and inhibitors tolerated, and thus purification steps not required
Detects DNA	Detects DNA and RNA
Tested on patient samples	Less tested on patient samples

It can be preserved in a lyophilized form which can be stored at a very low temperature (Klaster et al., 1998). The LAMP products can be detected by many approaches such as gel electrophoresis, optical devices or visual inspection, which showed high sensitivity and specificity, rapidness and cost-effectiveness (Ge et al., 2013; Marthaler et al., 2014; Yuan et al., 2014). Its positive reaction can be easily detected by the naked eye, since a large amount of white precipitate of magnesium pyrophosphate emerges in the reaction mixture (Mei et al., 2019). Other researchers also reported that LAMP products can easily be detected by the naked eye or by adding a variety of DNA-intercalating dyes to the tube, allowing researchers to observe the color change of the solution (Iwamoto et al., 2003; Tomita et al.,

2008; Ball et al., 2016). The LAMP method relies on auto-cycling strand displacement DNA synthesis by Bst DNA polymerase, with 4 or 6 primers recognizing 6-8 distinct regions of the target gene (Mori et al., 2001; Nagamine et al., 2001; Enosawa et al., 2003), which can be performed easily and quickly under isothermal conditions ranging from 60 °C to 65 °C for 30-60 minutes (Notomi et al., 2000; Mori et al., 2001; Enosawa et al., 2003; Tomita et al., 2008). In comparison with real-time PCR, the LAMP assay developed can provide a rapid and simple approach for routine screening and specific detection of GMOs (Liu et al., 2009; Feng et al., 2015; Tu et al., 2020), beer-spoilage microorganisms (Tsuchiya et al., 2007), malaria (Han, 2013; Zhang et al., 2017), and poultry pathogens (Ehtisham-Ul-Haque et al., 2018). LAMP based isothermal amplification of adenovirus genome for detection and typing of adenoviruses is farther than PCR based methods (Wakabayashi et al., 2004). LAMP for DNA amplification, detection is based on either turbidity (Fukuta et al., 2004; Huang et al., 2014), or SYBR Green I mediated fluorescence (Chen et al., 2012; Huang et al., 2014; Wang et al., 2015). LAMP product can be detected by electrophoresis, and it can be judged by white precipitate or color change (Focke et al., 2013; Deb et al., 2016). Reverse transcription loop-mediation isothermal amplification assay can be used as the basis for a rapid and low-cost assay for differentiation of foot-and-mouth disease (FMD) from other vesicular diseases in the field (Fowler et al., 2016). Lu et al., (2019) reported that a loop-mediated isothermal amplification with lateral flow dipstick (LAMP-LFD) method is an appropriate method for Bombyx mori bidensovirus (BmBDV) detection. LAMP methods have been applied to the detection of pork, chicken, bovine meat and ostrich meat (Ahmed et al., 2010; Abdulmawjood et al., 2014). Lee et al., (2019) reported that the portable LAMP device coupled with a syringe-filter based DNA extraction method enables us to detect the presence of fecal indicator bacteria (FIB) for assessing microbial water quality within 1 hour without any sophisticated laboratory equipment or highly trained personnel. Samples of loop-mediated amplification (LAMP) assay for rapid detection of the most important human and plant diseases are shown in Table 6. RT-LAMP assays for COVID-19 detection are shown in Table 7.

Table 6. Samples of loop-mediated isothermal amplification (LAMP) assay for rapid detection of the most important human and plant diseases

Disease	Rapid detection	Reference
Severe Acute Respiratory Syndrome (SARS-CoV)	a. The LAMP assay has been used for SARS-CoV	Hong et al., (2004)
Human coronavirus NL63	a. The LAMP assay does not cross-react with other respiratory viruses.	Pyrc et al., (2011)
Middle East Respiratory Syndrome (MERS-CoV)	a. A reverse transcription (RT)-LAMP assays using quenching probes (QProbes) for detection of MERS-COV has been confirmed.	Shirato et al., (2014) Bhadra et al., (2015) Lee et al., (2016) Shirato et al., (2018)
SARS-CoV-2	a. RT-LAMP assays have been evaluated using specimens collected from COVID-19 patients that exhibited high agreement to the qRT-PCR. b. mRT-LAMP coupled with a nanoparticle based lateral flow biosensor assay (mRT-LAMP-LFB) assay was successfully devised for detecting SARS-CoV-2 infection, which only requires simple heating equipment to maintain a constant temperature of 63oC for 40 min.	Baek et al., (2020) Kitagawa et al., (2020) Park et al., (2020) Yan et al., (2020) Zhu et al., (2020)
Influenza	a. RT-LAMP assay is a sensitive, rapid and specific method for the detection of Influenza. b. The assays are useful for experimental, hospital and quarantine laboratories.	Imai et al., (2006) Imai et al., (2007) Jayawardena et al., (2007) Ahn et al., (2019) Ma et al., (2019) Shi et al., (2019) Takayama et al., (2019) Thi et al., (2020)
Herpes simplex virus (HSV-1)	a. The LAMP assay is a rapid highly specific and sensitive method for the diagnosis of retinitis caused by HSV-1.	Reddy et al., (2011)
Cyprinid Herpes virus-3 (CyHV-3)	a. The combination of LAMP assay with the nucleic acid lateral flow analysis can simplify the diagnosis and screening of CyHV-3.	Soliman and El-Matbouli (2010)

Disease	Rapid detection	Reference
Malaria	a. The multiple microfluidic LAMP (mμLAMP) assay displayed high consistency with that by morphological analysis. b. LAMP method is robust for diagnosing malaria, both in symptomatic and asymptomatic people. The diagnostic odds ration of LAMP versus microscopy was >900.	Mao et al., (2018) Charpentier et al., (2020) Picot et al., (2020)
Dengue virus	a. RT-LAMP assay by newly designed primers for Dengue virus detection provides a facile and accurate molecular amplification technique for the rapid discriminative detection of dengue viruses.	Kim et al., (2018)
Tumor cells	a. A novel loop-mediated isothermal amplification (PA-LAMP) enables highly specific and sensitive single nucleotide mutation detection of genomic DNA in tumor cells.	Du et al., (2019)
Hepatitis B virus (HBV)	a. The final optimized fluorescence-based LAMP assay provided significant amplification time of less than 15 minutes compared with over 1 hour for PCR and opened tube LAMP system.	Quoc et al., (2018)
Zika virus	a. The novel ZikV RT-LAMP assays proved to have good performance and reliability.	Tian et al., (2016) Escalante-Maldonado et al., (2019)
Neurocysticercosis (NCC)	a. LAMP assay can detect DNA in blood. Real time LAMP assays for Tenia solium cox1 gene in blood helps in diagnosis of NCC. Its sensitivity and specificity of LAMP assay in NCC is 74% and 90%, respectively. Positive predictive value of LAMP assay in NCC is 93%.	Goyal et al., (2020)
Celiac disease (CD)	a. Combined with point-of-care antibody testing, CD-LAMP may enable immediate, confident CD diagnosis at a low cost in the clinical setting.	Erlichster et al., (2018)
HIV-1 infection	a. The RT-LAMP procedure was modified for the direct detection of HIV-1 nucleic acid in plasma and blood samples, eliminating the need for an additional nucleic acid extraction step and reducing the overall procedure time to approximately 90 min.	Curtis et al., (2008)
Toxoplasma gondii	a. It is a major parasite of warm-blooded animals including man. LAMP technique was superior to PCR in detecting the murine *Toxoplasma* infection.	Hegazy et al., (2020)
Helicobacter pylori	a. The LAMP assay was highly sensitive, rapid and simple for *Helicobacter pylori* cagA gene, and *H. pylori* infections.	Horiuchi et al., (2019)
Pectobacterium atrosepticum	a. The LAMP assay differentiates *P. atrosepticum* from other pectolytic potato pathogens and other bacteria.	Li et al., (2011)
Pectobacterium carotovorum	a. It is the causal agent of bacterial soft rot in a wide range of vegetable host species. A LAMP assay, in conjunction with a crude DNA extraction method, was successfully performed on *P. carotovorum*-infected samples derived from both artificially and naturally infected plants.	Shi et al., (2020)

Table 6. (Continued)

Disease	Rapid detection	Reference
Pythium insidiosum	a. It causes a life-threatening condition called pythiosis. LAMP is a suitable and efficient assay for detecting *P. insidiosum* infection in the resource-limited laboratories.	Htun et al., (2020)
Duck hepatitis B virus (DHBV)	a. The LAMP method has the advantage of simplicity, high sensitivity and specificity, good visibility, low cost and is more practical and convenient than PCR-related assays for the clinical detection of DHBV.	Jun et al., (2020)
Pyrenochaeta lycopersici	a. The LAMP method showed equal sensitivity to polymerase chain reaction in molecular identification of the pathogen in cultured mycelia, infested plant roots, and their surrounding soil.	Hienko et al., (2016)
Lymphocystis disease virus (LDV)	a. It has potential for early diagnosis of LDV because of its suitability and simplicity of the test.	Li et al., (2010)
Swine acute diarrhea syndrome coronavirus (SADS-CoV)	a. A novel real-time RT-LAMP method was developed for detection of SADS-CoV in pigs.	Wang et al., (2018)
Swine vesicular disease virus (SVDV)	a. One-step reverse transcriptase loop-mediated isothermal amplification (RT-LAMP) assay is sensitive, rapid, and the isothermal amplification strategy used is not reliant on expensive equipment.	Blomstrom et al., (2008)
Classical swine fever virus (CSFV)	a. The RT-LAMP assay can be used for rapid laboratory diagnosis and pen-side detection for CSFV detection in pigs.	Yin et al., (2010)
African Swine Fever (ASF)	a. ASFV-LAMP assay and hue-saturation-value (HSV) color space transformation may accelerate the screening process of pigs for ASFV infection. b. The LAMP assays were comparable to the well-established real-time PCR assay.	Yu et al., (2020) Wang et al., (2020)
Porcine circovirus 3 (PCV-3)	a. The LAMP assay using HNB was developed for the rapid and visual detection of PCV-3.	Park et al., (2018)
Avian bornavirus (ABV)	a. RT-LAMP assay has 100 times higher sensitivity than that or RT-qPCR for screening and field surveys of ABV-infected birds.	Komorizono et al., (2020)
Infectious bursal disease virus (IBDV)	a. RT-LAMP combined with a chromatographic lateral flow dipstick (LFD) is appropriate for the detection of IBDV.	Tsai et al., (2012)

Disease	Rapid detection	Reference
Marek's disease virus (MDV)	a. LAMP assay is a sensitive, rapid and specific method for the detection of MDV.	Wei et al., (2012)
Human papillomaviruses (HPV)	a. LAMP has an overall sensitivity of 99.4% and specificity of 93.2% relative to PCR which has made it a promising technology for accurate diagnosis of high-risk HPV infection.	Livingstone et al., (2016) Yang et al., (2016)
Burkholderia mallei	a. LAMP assay being simple and rapid can be a viable alternative to PCR-based glanders diagnostic assays in glanders endemic regions.	Saxena et al., (2019)
Vibrio parahaemolyticus	a. Combining LAMP and disposable electrochemical sensors based on screen printed grapheme electrodes (SPGEs) is suitable as a point-of-care device for on-site detection of food-borne pathogens.	Pasookhush et al., (2016) Kampeera et al., (2019) Lee et al., (2020)
Infectious bronchitis virus (IBV)	a. Reverse-transcription LAMP (RT-LAMP) has been used as a qualitative detection tool.	Wu et al., (2019)
Newcastle disease virus (NDV)	a. Reverse-transcription LAMP (RT-LAMP) has been used as a qualitative detection tool.	Wu et al., (2019)
Morganella morganii	a. Improved LAMP assay could significantly distinguish *M. morganii* from other bacteria.	Shahbazi et al., (2019)
Phytophthora infestans	a. LAMP-*P. infestans* specific multiple copy DNA sequences (PiSMC) assay is available for early diagnosis of potato late blight.	Kong et al., (2020)
Phytophthora capsici	a. The detection limit of *P. capsici* LAP was 100 fg genomic DNA per 25 μL reaction.	Dong et al., (2015)
Andrias davidianus	a. LAMP assay is used for rapid detection of the Chinese giant salamander iridovirus (GSIV) infection.	Meng et al., (2013)
Sacbrood virus (SBV)	a. LAMP-based assay is a useful tool for the rapid and sensitive diagnosis of Chinese sacbrood virus (CSBV) infection of bees.	Ma et al., (2011)
T gene of Aves polyomavirus I (APyV)	a. LAMP assay is a valuable tool for the rapid, sensitive and specific detection of APyV from budgerigar fledgling disease (BFD)-suspected psittacine bird samples.	Park et al., (2019)
Helicobacter pylori	a. LAMP can be used for diagnosing and screening of *H. pylori* infections to decrease gastric cancer incidence.	Horiuchi et al., (2019)
Beak and feather disease virus (BFDV)	a. Swarm primer-applied loop-mediated isothermal amplification (sLAMP) is a valuable tool for rapid, sensitive, specific and reliable detection of BFDV.	Kuo et al., (2015) Chae et al., (2020)

Table 6. (Continued)

Disease	Rapid detection	Reference
Foot-and-mouth disease virus (FMDV)	a. RT-LAMP chemistry with multiple sample types, both in the presence and absence of nucleic acid extraction, provides advantages over alternative isothermal chemistries and alternative pen-side diagnostics such as antigen-detection lateral-flow devices.	Guan et al., (2013) Yamazaki et al., (2013) Ding et al., (2014) Waters et al., (2014) Howson et al., (2015) Howson et al., (2017)
Bovine popular stomatitis virus (BPSV)	a. The LAMP assay for BPSV was developed which was similarly sensitive as semi-nested PCR assay for parapoxvirus.	Kurosaki et al., (2016)
Lawsonia intracellularis	a. LAMP assay could be a useful alternative tool in point-of-care (POC) diagnosis of *L. intracellularis* infection.	Li et al., (2018)
Hepatocellular carcinoma	a. RT-LAMP is a rapid, sensitive and economic way for the rapid identification of cancer stem cell-specific biomarkers to estimate the potential risk of HCC metastasis.	Yao et al., (2020)
Streptococcus pyogenes	a. The rapid detection of the streptococcal pyrogenic exotoxin B (speB) gene by the LAMP assay is both sensitive and specific.	Cao et al., (2016)
Streptococcus mutans	a. LAMP has been used for the rapid detection of cnm-positive *S. mutans* associated with cerebral microhemorrhage. This method resulted in a cnm-positive rate of 26.4% in 102 samples, which was higher than that obtained with conventional PCR.	Kitagawa et al., (2020)
Dracunculus medinensis	a. A LAMP test was developed to amplify DNA from copepods to use as an internal amplification control during testing. b. Results are achieved in less than 30 min using just the Genie III instrument and no other laboratory equipment is necessary.	Boonham et al., (2020)
Trypanosoma evansi	a. This infection (Surra) is one of the most important diseases of camels in North and East Africa. A novel dry LAMP is developed which diagnoses *Trypanosoma evansi* infection targeting the RoTat1.2 VSG gene.	Salim et al., (2018)
Mycobacterium marinum	a. It is an aquatic pathogenic species. The LAMP system was established for detection of *M. marinum* which showed high sensitivity and specificity for its detection.	Tsai et al., (2019)
Horse meat	a. Detection of horse DNA by LAMP is a promising detection method.	Aartse et al., (2017)

Disease	Rapid detection	Reference
Bovine herpesvirus-1 (BoHV-1)	a. The LAMP method is a potential tool for rapid, sensitive, specific, cost-effective, and user-friendly detection and differentiation of wild type BoHV-1 from gE-deleted marker vaccine.	Parwar et al., (2015)
Feline infectious peritonitis (FIP)	a. Although the RT-LAMP assay is less sensitive than real time reverse transcription PCR (RT-PCR), it can be performed without the need of expensive equipment with less hands-on time.	Gunther et al., (2018)
Salmonella strains	a. A developed visual loop-mediated isothermal amplification combined with lateral flow dipstick (LAMP-LFD) method targeting the hilA gene is a promising detection method for *Salmonella*. b. Direct triplex LAMP could detect *Salmonella* at 6.4 × 101 CFU/g in chicken meat, which could be utilized for point-of-care testing in various industries.	Kumar et al., (2014) Hu et al., (2018) Mei et al., (2019) Kim et al., (2021)
Halichoerus grypus	a. LAMP assay offers the possibility to confirm injuries that have been caused by a grey seal.	Heers et al., (2018)
Porphyromonas gingivalis	a. MB-LAMP (molecular beacon-Loop-mediated isothermal amplification) is a rapid and sensitive assay developed to diagnose *P. gingivalis*.	Liu et al., (2017) Su et al., (2019)
Peronophythora litchii	a. It is one of the most destructive of lychee and LAMP assay is able to detect *P. litchii* in plant tissues and soils. The optimal LAMP assay was established based on the sequence of *P. litchi* M90 gene.	Kong et al., (2021)
Milk vetch dwarf virus (MDV)	a. The LAMP method is recommended for the detection of MDV.	Zhang et al., (2018)
Lactobacillus crispatus	a. The LAMP assay had a lower limit of detection of 10 fg DNA and could detect it within 45 minutes.	Higashide et al., (2019)
Lactobacillus iners	a. The LAMP assay had a lower limit of detection of 10 fg DNA and could detect it within 45 minutes.	Higashide et al., (2019)
Nosema ceranae	a. LAMP gave good results and it could be an alternative diagnostic tool instead of PCR to detect *N. ceranae* infection in honeybee.	Chupia et al., (2016)
Banna virus (BAV)	a. A rapid, sensitive and specific RT-LAMP assay can be applied for BAV detection in clinical or field samples.	Xia et al., (2019)
Aspergillus species	a. The assay combined with a suitable protocol for in field crude DNA extraction and a colorimetric method is a reliable tool to support reduction strategies of mycotoxin contamination in crop management programs.	Ferrara et al., (2020)
Karenia mikimotoi	a. LAMP in combination with the lateral flow dipstick (LFD) is appropriate for rapid field detection of low density *K. mikimotoi* and early prevention of red tide induced by such algae.	Huang et al., (2020)

Table 6. (Continued)

Disease	Rapid detection	Reference
Chattonella marina	a. The established LAMP products by lateral-flow dipstick displayed good specificity and no cross reaction was detected with non-target algal species.	Qin et al., (2019)
Klebsiella pneumoniae carbapenemases (KPC)	a. The LAMP assay may be routinely applied for detection of KPC producers in the clinical laboratory.	Nakano et al., (2015)
Mycoplasma genitalium	a. The LAMP assay was designed to detect the pdhD gene of genomic DNA.	Edwards et al., (2015)
Mycobacterium tuberculosis	a. LAMP system has the potential to be a point of care test for early diagnosis of active tuberculosis.	Thapa et al., (2019)
Rhizoctonia solani	a. The LAMP-LFD detected *R. solani* in infected plant tissues, samples, seeds, vegetative cuttings and soil samples.	Patel et al., (2015)
Vibrio parahaemolyticu	a. LAMP has emerged as a potential tool for the detection of *V. parahaemolyticus*.	Anupama et al., (2019 Xing et al., (2020)
Vibrio alginolyticus	a. The LAMP-LFD method targeted to the rpoX gene is a convenient assay for specific identification of *V. alginolyticus* with high sensitivity.	Plaon et al., (2015)
Vibrio cholera O1 and O139	a. Multiple LAMP-based methods for rapid detection of cholera causing agents were developed.	Izumiya et al., (2019)
Pepper mottle virus (PepMoV)	a. RT-LAMP assay could be a useful alternative tool for the diagnosis and epidemiological surveillance of PepMoV infections.	Luo et al., (2016)
Pepper vein yellows virus (PeVYV)	a. PeVYV-specific RT-LAMP assay is recommended for large scale field studies of PeVYV infection.	Jiang et al., (2017)
Potato virus a (PVA)	a. RT-LAMP assay was used for the detection of PVA from potato tubers. The SP-RT-LAMP was successful in the detection of PVA in single aphids.	Raigond et al., (2020)
Tobacco streak virus (TSV)	a. The RT-LAMP diagnostic tool can be utilized for rapid detection of TSV in cotton.	Gawande et al., (2019)
Abaca bunchy top virus (ABTV)	a. LAMP primers were designed to detect ABTV. LAMP protocols can detect ABTV up to 0.01 fg, which is more sensitive and faster than PCR.	Galvez et al., (2020)
Sugarcane mosaic disease (SMD)	a. The RT-LAMP assay is highly specific in discriminating sugarcane mosaic disease virus from viral pathogens of sugarcane, which is about 10-fold more sensitive than conventional RT-PCR.	Wang et al., (2019)

Disease	Rapid detection	Reference
Fusarium spp.	a. LAMP primers binding to FUM1 gene were designed for potential fumonisin producers, which can be a versatile tool that targets the reduction of fumonisins in the food and feed chain.	Wigmann et al., (2020)
Fusarium proliferatum	a. The LAMP assay could be suitable for diagnosis of ear and kernel rot on maize caused by *F. proliferatum*. b. TEF-1α region is appropriate for LAMP primers that are highly specific for it. SYBR Green I is found to be an indicator for the rapid and practical diagnostics of LAMP assay.	Wang et al., (2020)
Fusarium temperatum	a. It is an emerging pathogen and represents a toxicological risk to maize from pre-harvest to storage stage. A visualized LAMP assay for its rapid diagnosis was developed.	Shan et al., (2019)
Dusarium oxysporum f.sp. melonis	a. The LAMP is a simple reliable tool for diagnosing fusarium wilt of melon.	Almasi (2019)
Bean common mosaic necrosis virus (BCMNV)	a. LAMP primer set for the detection of BCMNV was developed which is more rapid and specific in leguminous crops than conventional RT-nested PCR method.	Lee et al., (2017)
Mesta yellow vein mosaic virus (MeYVMV)	a. LAMP assay developed for the detection of MeYVMV in mesta is more sensitive than PCR technique. b. LAMP assay has been optimized using Hydroxy Naphthol Blue (HNB) dye which is more suitable for field sample diagnosis and in quarantine.	Meena et al., (2019)
Maize chlorotic mottle virus in maize (MCMV)	a. The RT-LAMP could be completed within 60 min using the primers designed in the CP gene. It was about 10-fold more sensitive than RT-PCR.	Chen et al., (2017)
Turnip yellows virus (TuYV)	a. The RT-LAMP assay protocol enables quicker and cheaper diagnosis for TuYV than current techniques. b. It has potential for earlier in-field detection in combination with aphid trapping programs.	Congdon et al., (2019)
Citrus leaf blotch virus (CLBV)	a. The sensitivity of RT-LAMP method was increased 100-fold compared to that of the conventional RT-PCR.	Liu et al., (2019)
Onion yellow dwarf virus (OYDV)	a. RT-LAMP assay could be used in plant pathology laboratories with limited facilities and resources as well as directly in the field.	Tiberini et al., (2019)
Little cherry virus 1 (LChV-1)	a. The LChV-1-specific RT-LAMP reaction can be completed within 10 min. Its sensitivity assay was up to 100x higher than conventional RT-PCR assays.	Tahzima et al., (2019)
Genetically modified organisms (GMOs)	a. LAMP-mediated novel, comprehensive and rapid detection methods for GM maize and soybean events were developed. b. LAMP facilitates on-site GM detection if combined with fast DNA extraction method.	Li et al., (2018) Takabatake et al., (2018) Singh et al., (2019)

Table 7. RT-LAMP assays for COVID-19 detection

RT-LAMP assays	Key points	Reference
Rapid detection with RT-LAMP	a. A rapid screening LAMP test for COVID-19 with an assay time under 30 min was reported.	Lamb et al., (2020)
Rapid RT-LAMP for ORF1ab, S gene and N gene	a. 4 sets of LAMP primers which targeted different gene regions of COVID-19 were designed. b. Two primer sets (N1 and N15) target the N gene of the virus, while the other two (S17 and O117) target the S gene and ORF1ab gene of SARS-CoV-2, respectively. c. The ORF1ab gene targeted is close to the 5/-end of the viral RNA, while the N gene is close to the 3/-end.	Huang et al., (2020)
iLACO (Isothermal LAMP based method for COVID-19) assay	a. iLACO assay was developed to target an ORF1ab gene for molecular diagnosis of the novel coronavirus. b. The iLACO was vastly faster than the conventional PCR method due to its high amplification efficiency. c. The iLACO detection process takes 15-40 min, depending on the viral load in the sample.	Yu et al., (2020a,b)
One-pot RT-LAMP assay	a. One-pot RT-LAMP assays were developed in order to detect the N gene of COVID-19 with simplicity. b. It was concluded that was best to use 5 μL of blood sample volume for a 50 μL reaction, as it is the highest sample volume added that still showed acceptable amplification of nucleic acid.	Wang (2020)
Mismatch-Tolerant RT-LAMP	a. One way implementation of mismatch-tolerant LAMP assay, which can be realized through the addition of 0.15 U of high-fidelity DNA polymerase may increase the quality and reliability of the detection results. b. When compared to a commercial RT-1PCR assay with 24 clinical samples, the novel RT-LAMP assay showed 100% consistency, validating that this assay can detect COVID-19 RNA as reliably as RT-PCR method.	Lu et al., (2020) Thompson and Lei (2020)
Barcoded RT-LAMP (LAMP-Seq)	a. A barcoded RT-LAMP procedure called LAMP-Seq was developed in order to detect COVID-19 on a large scale. b. In a typical detection protocol, wab sample is first added to a RT-LAMp reaction, which contains the 6 different LAMP primers targeting the N gene, and the forward inner primer (FIP) is barcoded with a compressed barcode space of 10 nucleotides in order to label the specific sample for identification.	Schmid-Burgk et al., (2020)
Sample inactivation and purification for RT-LAMP	a. Unique sample preparation steps can be added to LAMP assays in order to increase sensitivity of the assay, while also increasing the stability of the viral RNA samples and lowering the risks of handling of the infectious virus.	Rabe and Cepko (2020)

RT-LAMP assays	Key points	Reference
Penn-RAMP	a. Penn-RAMP is a novel single and two-stage isothermal amplification assay which was developed to target the ORF1ab gene of viral RNA with enhanced performance. b. In comparison of the three methods (COVID-19 Penn-RAMP, COVID-19 LAMP, and COVID-19 RT-PCR) using synthetic COVID-19 sequences, it was observed that the novel Penn-RAMP method is the best diagnostic procedure. c. Unlike RT-PCR and similar to RT-LAMP assays, it is conducted at isothermal conditions, so the overall costs of operation are reduced. It has also the greatest activity and high sensitivity.	El-Tholoth et al., (2020) Thompson and Lei (2020)
Integrated RT-LAMP and CRISPR-Cas 12 method	a. The novel CRISPR-enabled detection method, called COVID-19 DNA Endonuclease-Targeted CRISPR Trans Reporter (DETECTR), utilizes a Cas12 enzyme after an RT-LAMP procedure to detect a specific E gene and N gene sequence in the amplified virus RNA and indiscriminately cleave nearby structures once complexed.	Broughton et al., (2020)
SHERLOCK with integrated RT-LAMP	a. The integrated RT-LAMP and SHERLOCK (specific high sensitivity enzymatic reporter unlocking) process consists of isothermal amplification of viral RNA and sequential detection of amplicon from CRISPR-mediated reporter cleaving.	Joung et al., (2020)

Chapter 9

Rapid Disease Detection

There are numerous rapid antigen detection testing methods, namely latex agglutination, enzyme immunoassay, optical immunoassay, chemiluminescent DNA probes and PCR methods (Leung et al., 2006; Akhtar and Stern, 2012). The rapid detection of resistance is a challenge for clinical microbiologists who wish to prevent deleterious individual and collective consequences (Decousser et al., 2017). Nested PCR assay is more sensitive than immunocytochemical (IFL) for the detection of *Pneumocystis carinii* in AIDS patients, prior to the debut of PCR symptoms (Olsson et al., 1996). Immunochromatography assays (ICA) have proven to be a rapid, simple, effective and economical method for the detection of *Pseudomonas aeruginosa* infection in clinical samples (Wang et al., 2011). Group B streptococci (GBS) specific PCR assays using real-time PCR and fluorescence labeling technologies offer promising tools for sensitive and specific detection of GBS directly from clinical specimens (Ke and Bergeron, 2001). Monoclonal antibodies with inhibition effect have been utilized for the synchronous detection of three avian influenza antibodies in different species (Xiao et al., 2019). Swarm primer-applied loop-mediated isothermal amplification assay is a valuable tool for rapid, sensitive, specific and reliable detection of beak and feather disease virus (BFDV) in suspected psittacine birds (Chae et al., 2020). Xiong et al., (2019) concluded that the proposed one-step competitive immunoassay has great potential applications in the rapid laboratory diagnosis of Wilson's disease (WD) with distinct advantages. Two-step reverse transcription recombinase polymerase amplification assay combined with lateral flow detection (RPA-LFD) was recognized as an appropriate method to detect foot-and moth disease virus (FMDV) (Wang et al., 2018a). A direct double antibody lateral flow assay (DDA-gB-LFA) provides a rapid, sensitive, and specific detection of Aujeszky's disease virus (ADV) glycoprotein B (gB)-directed antibodies in sera and can be used for the detection of ADV-exposed swine (Vrublevskaya et al., 2017). A deep-red fluorogenic probe (BT-NH) could be a potential biological fluorogenic tool to explore the roles of Nitric oxide (NO) in Parkinson's disease (PD) (Weng et al., 2019). For viral infectious diseases, molecular diagnostic testing, the detection of viral DNAs or RNAs from infected patients, remains the gold standard (Speers, 2006; Souf, 2016). Zheng and Huo (2020) reported a new rapid blood test for virus infection detection and diagnosis such as ongoing COVID-19. Reverse transcription strand invasion based amplification (RT-SIBA) assay was a rapid molecular assay for the detection of respiratory syncytial virus (RSV) with good performance in clinical specimens (Eboigbodin et al., 2017; Alidjinou et al., 2019).

Magnetic-quantum dot nanobead can serve as enrichment substrate and fluorescent probe for virus detection using lateral flow assay (Bai et al., 2020). Biosensors provided highly sensitive and selective detection of influenza virus (Hassanpour et al., 2018). Rapid diagnostic tests for infectious diseases, with a turnaround time of less than 2 hours, are promising tools that could improve patient care, antimicrobial stewardship and infection prevention in the emergency department setting (Bouzid et al., 2020). The novel biosensor platform demonstrates good stability and selectivity which can be implemented for point-of-care diagnosis of biomarkers related to other infectious diseases (Paul et al., 2017). Quartz crystal microbalance (QCM)-based biosensors are promising tools for the rapid detection of infections, and microfluidic systems can boost the applicability of QCM for point-of-care diagnosis (Lim et al., 2020). Genosensor is based on a very simple methodology which can be followed based on its easy-to-access approach and it is quick and could be used as a point-of-care test for the detection of influenza virus within 30 min (Ravina et al., 2020). Nishiyama et al., (2020) reported a rapid, facile and selective detection of anti-H5 subtype avian influenza virus antibody in serum by fluorescence polarization immunoassay (FPIA). Novel, low cost and easy to use Q-tips colorimetric biosensor assay for flue A and B viruses was developed, where the Q-tips swab serves as sample collection, analytes pre-concentration as well as sensing tool (Raji et al., 2021). The pyrosequencing assay is highly sensitive, robust and provides a rapid assay suitable for detecting influenza B variants in respiratory clinical specimens or isolates (Lau et al., 2019). Combining saliva and nasophayngeal swabs (NPS) could improve the sensitivities of influenza rapid influenza diagnostic tests (RIDTs) (Yoon et al., 2017). It is essential to define diagnostic performance of rapid influenza detection kits (Chan et al., 2012). Daum et al., (2002) reported that RT-PCR assay is a highly sensitive and timely surveillance tool for rapid detection and simultaneous subtyping of clinical influenza specimens isolated worldwide. Novel TaqMan RT-PCR assay for detection of the influenza A (H2) viruses was designed, and designed primers and probes used for the real-time RT-PCR universal detection of influenza A viruses could be used in clinical trials of vaccines against influenza A and screening for H2 in cases of unsubtypeable influenza A in humans (Komissarov et al., 2017). Jokela et al., (2015) reported that Alere I Influenza A&B assay is a good alternative to rapid immunochromatographic tests.

Chapter 10

PCR and Epidemic Diseases

PCR technology has emerged as a basic tool in biological research and in the detection of infectious organisms and can provide information on a number of toxins and virulence factors (Singh et al., 2003). The application of multiplex PCR for the detection of multiple pathogens within the same sample will provide a major contribution to the efficiency, logistics and cost-effectiveness of molecular diagnostics (Molenkamp et al., 2007). The mRT-PCR is a useful tool for epidemiological studies and laboratory diagnosis of single virus and mixed infections in swine (Zhao et al., 2019). Kost (2018) reported molecular detection and point-of-care testing of Ebola virus disease and other threats. Real time PCR may provide a rapid, specific method which enables detection and characterization of infectious laryngotracheitis virus (ILTV) directly from field cases (Creelan et al., 2006).

Some techniques employing nucleic acid-based assays have essential roles in monitoring the spread of West Nile virus (Shi and Kramer, 2003). RT-PCR has been used during gastroenteritis epidemic outbreak (Jothikumar et al., 1994), and could simplify early plant disease diagnosis and assist in monitoring the dissemination of the pathogen within and between fields (Araujo et al., 2007). A duplex real-time RT-PCR assay is a powerful tool for studies of Borna disease virus (BDV), including epidemiological screening and diagnosis (Wensman et al., 2007), and it can also exhibit higher sensitivity than virus isolation and could be used for rapid diagnosis of infectious bronchitis virus (IBV) in the field (Ramneek et al., 2005). RT-PCR assays have been reported as a promising method for detection and differentiation of all major types of US porcine epidemic diarrhea virus (PEDV) variants (Liu and Wang, 2016). Bachanek-Bankowska et al., (2016) recommended serotype-special real-time RT-PCR assay for detection and characterization of foot-and-mouth disease virus (FMDVs). Maurin (2012) found that real-time PCR tests are well-suited for the rapid detection of bacteria directly in clinical specimens, allowing early, sensitive and specific laboratory confirmation of related diseases. Molecular PCR-based strategies are best for the targeted screening of complex biological environments (Decousser et al., 2017). Klingspor and Jalal (2006) reported that the real-time PCR assay allows sensitive and specific detection and identification of fungal pathogens in vitro and in vivo. Two important PCR methods used in laboratory diagnosis of respiratory viruses are conventional PCR, which is usually evaluated by colorometry or agarose gel electrophoresis, and real-time PCR, and multiplex PCR (Olofsson et al., 2011). A real-time quantitative fluorescence polymerase chain reaction (QF-PCR) method has high sensitivity, specificity, and repeatability, and provides reliable technological support for the detection, prevention and control of *Mycoplasma mycoides* subsp. Capri (Mmc) infection (Lin et al., 2019). PCR based molecular approaches are independent of antibiotic, more rapid, reliable and sensitive and can be routinely used as molecular tools for pathogen identification (Clarridge and Jill, 2004). Quantitative real-time PCR is much less time and labor intensive than conventional PCR since there is computerized evaluation of positive and negative results as well as computerized generation of quantitative data (Schuler and Dolken, 2006). Vendittelli et al., (2015) demonstrated the usefulness of multimarker qRT-PCR to detect circulating melanoma cells in blood and for potentially assessing patient disease status or progression. The selection of both the human clinical specimen and the reverse transcriptase enzyme involved in the molecular detection of Zika virus (ZIKV) by quantitative real-time polymerase chain reaction (qRT-PCR) played an important role in enabling improved detection of the virus (Viedma et al., 2019). Burchard et al., (2014) developed a comprehensive RT-PCR, easy-to-use assay for the detection of HIV-1 in human plasma. Liu et al., (2011) showed that multiplex RT-PCR provides a new assay for rapid detection and differentiation of both classes of Newcastle disease isolates. Horwood and Mahony (2011) observed a real-time PCR method for BPIV-3 and the first multiplex designed to detect three bovine respiratory disease complex (BRDC) viral pathogens. A simple and fast sap-direct RT-PCR is considered as an effective method for the identification and cloning of *coleus blumei* viroids (CbVds) (Jiang et al., 2011). Zhao et al., (2014) reported that the multiplex TaqMan probe-based real-time PCR should be a useful tool for quantifying viral load, detecting porcine epidemic diarrhea virus (PEDV), and differentiating variant from classical PEDV. The multiplex PCR (mPCR) assay represented an economical, reproducible and robust diagnostic tool for concurrent detection of cattle haemoparasites and large scale epidemiological studies (Ganguly et al., 2020). Wang et al., (2014) and He et al., (2019) also reported a duplex real-time RT-PCR assay for detection and differentiation of the variant and the virulent strains of PEDV currently circulating. The SYBR Green real-time RT-PCR assay is more sensitive than conventional RT-PCR and nested PCR assays, and has potential as a reliable, reproductive, specific, sensitive and rapid tool for detection, quantitation and diagnosis of unclassified bovine enteric calicivirus (BECV) (Park et al., 2009). Lymphocystis disease virus (LCDV) qPCR assays are highly sensitive, specific, reproducible and versatile for the detection and quantitation of *Lymphocystivirus*, and may also be used for asymptomatic carrier detection or pathogenesis studies of different LCDV strains (Ciulli et al., 2015). Wilkes et al., (2015) reported that insulated isothermal PCR (iiPCR) technology has potential to serve as a useful tool for rapid and accurate points of need, molecular detection of CPV-2. Thanthrige-Don et al., (2018) introduced multiplex PCR-electronic microarray assay for screening of healthy animals to identify carriers that may potentially develop bovine respiratory disease complex (BRDC) and bovine enteric disease (BED). Wu et al., (2017) reported that RT-droplet digital PCR (ddPCR) assay could be used as an efficient molecular biology tool to diagnose Japanese encephalitis virus (JEV) which would be beneficial for public health security. The duplex PCR has been recognized as a useful tool for *Erysipelothrix rhusiopathiae* infections' differential diagnosis in China (Zhu et al., 2017). Duplex conventional PCR is also useful for Las detection and identification for plant health certification and control program (Donnua et al., 2012). The duplex PCR assay could be a useful tool for hospital and veterinary surveillance studies on *Yersinia* worldwide (Rusak et al., 2018), and a sensitive and rapid method for the detection of porcine reproductive and respiratory syndrome virus (PRRSV) and porcine circovirus 2 (PCV-2) co-infection (Zheng et al., 2020).

Chapter 11

PCR and COVID-19

Poon et al., (2003) and Adachi et al., (2004) noted that by optimizing RNA extraction methods and applying quantitative real time RT-PCR technologies, the sensitivity of tests for early diagnosis of SARS can be greatly enhanced. The multiplex PCR technique could be applied to detect the SARS-CoV specific target cDNA fragments successfully (Chen et al., 2004; Yam et al., 2005). The PCR-based first test for diagnosis of COVID-19 was constructed in Germany; at first, before the release of sequence, RT-PCR assay was designed following SARS or SARS-like coronavirus because it was supposed that 2019-nCoV is SARS-related (Jalandra et al., 2020; Lv et al., 2020). Corman et al., (2020) developed a detection method that can differentiate between SARS-CoV and SARS-CoV-2, and they just selected two assays where E gene assay works as first-line screening tool and RdRp gene assay was done for confirmation of this testing. Wang (2020) supported the advantages of combination of Wantai Total Antibody assay and RT-PCR test for detection of SARS-CoV-2 infections. Double-quencher probes decreased the background fluorescence and improved the detection sensitivity of RT-PCR for SARS-CoV-2 (Hirotsu et al., 2020). Lv et al., (2020) observed that ddPCR has an advantage over qRT-PCR in tracing laboratory contamination. Attwood et al., (2020) recommended AusDiagnostics multiplex tandem PCR as a reliable tool for detection of COVID-19 virus. Boutin et al., (2020) demonstrated an excellent concordance between a laboratory developed RT-PCR and the cobas SARS-CoV-2 tests on the 8800 platform. Zou et al., (2020) indicated that the heat inactivation treatment before detection would reduce detection rates of SARS-CoV-2 in weakly positive clinical samples by qualitative real-time RT-PCR.

Chapter 12

Advantages and Disadvantages of Molecular Detection

Rapid and accurate diagnostic testing is an important step in diagnosing infectious diseases and determining the optimum approach to treatment and management. The most important advantages of molecular methodologies are sensitivity, specificity, turnaround time and application. Its sensitivity is related to identification of target molecules of interest that are only present in low concentrations. Its specificity minimizes and decreases false positive test results by targeting the specific molecule of interest. Molecular methodologies usually offer better and clear turnaround times from receipt to result reporting. Broader applications can be found with molecular methodologies such as infectious diseases, genetic testing, forensics, drug resistance and tumor marker detection and monitoring. The most important advantages of PCR tests are that they are useful in detecting cases of extra pulmonary specimens which may be missed by smear and culture, that they are a valuable method for detecting specific pathogens which are difficult to culture in vitro or require a long cultivation period, they are more rapid in providing results compared to culturing which consists of enabling earlier informed decision making, they enable rapid diagnosis of bacteremia, particularly for low levels of bacteria in specimens, and PCR is a valuable screening tool which is considered an adjunct test for certain diagnostic tests that reply on smear and culture (Wassenegger, 2001). Limitations of PCR testing are that PCR testing alone may be limited as a diagnostic tool, which still needs culture for testing for drug and antibiotic susceptibility and genetic typing; challenges of post treatment diagnosis which means that PCR detects dead organisms that may be shed for weeks after the patient stops showing symptoms; and that PCR results should be interpreted by a trained professional and they should not be used as the sole basis of patient treatment management decisions (Choe et al., 2015). PCR reliability, in terms of specificity of pathogen detection and quantification, has been improved by the use of sye quenched probes (Bonnet et al., 1999; Morris et al., 1996; Thelwell et al., 2000). The high sensitivity of the PCR can improved with the application of reverse-transcription-PCR (RT-PCR) (Lauri and Mariani, 2008), which requires the reverse-transcription of RNA by random primers and an RNA dependent DNA polymerase enzyme called reverse transcriptase. The resulting DNA copy of the RNA (cDNA) is used as template in the PCR (Lauri and Mariani, 2008). So far, RT-PCR has been mostly used to detect retroviruses, such as HIV, norovirus or avian influenza virus (Ngazoa et al., 2008). PCR does have its limitations because of false-negative and false-positive results which may be encountered with the daily running of PCR assays by a diagnostic laboratory (Maurer, 2010). A negative result means that there is no evidence of DNA or RNA of the target organism in the specimen tested. If no other etiology is identified and a specific infection is clinically suspected, additional specimens should be collected and tested. A positive result indicates detection of DNA or RNA and confirms infection, but does not necessarily mean a viable organism of interest is presented or that the patient is contagious. Potential advantages and disadvantages of molecular tests are shown in Table 8.

Table 8. Potential advantages and disadvantages of molecular tests

Potential advantages of molecular tests		**Potential disadvantages of molecular tests**	
a.	Increased sensitivity.	a.	Non-targeted organisms are not detected.
b.	Increased specificity, particularly for organisms with similar morphologies.	b.	Lack of standardization amongst laboratory-developed methods.
c.	Ability to differentiate species and strains beyond what is possible by morphology.	c.	High complexity testing.
d.	Not negatively influenced by altered or poor morphology.	d.	Requires expensive and sophisticated equipment.
		e.	Potential for nucleic and contamination.
		f.	Possible amplification inhibitors.
		g.	May not be performed rapidly.
		h.	Presence of DNA does not necessarily indicate active or symptomatic infection.

The most important advantages of molecular assay on the basis of PCR are that they are fully automated, that integrated devices run with single-use amplification test cartridges, that reagents for cartridges are freeze-dried and can be stored at room temperature, that some devices come with rechargeable batteries, that multiplex PCR can be used to detect several resistance markers at once, they have a quick turn-around time, they are a very reliable, known and trusted technology; and the most important disadvantages are that stand-alone assays require laboratory equipment, cartridges are expensive, devices require training in molecular laboratory techniques, devices are sensitive to ambient temperature and they require a constant energy supply to retain accuracy and function. False positives and false negative results of PCR are presented in Table 9.

Table 9. False positives and false negative results of PCR

False positives results	False negative results
1. Detecting contaminants introduced during specimen collection, transport or processing	1. Improper sample collection/transport
2. Detecting organisms representative of normal flora near specimen collection site, acid fast bacilli in water and contaminants in lab	2. Insufficient amount of specimen
3. Mislabeling	3. Degradation of nucleic acids (typically RNA) during storage and shipping
4. Specimen mix-up	4. Specimen collected prior to onset of symptoms or later in illness
	5. Quantity of organisms is below detection limit
	6. Non-homogeneous distribution of the organism of interest
	7. Presence of amplification inhibitors in the specimen
	8. Laboratory processing/testin errors

Table 10. The most important disadvantages of LAMP

a.	Most detection methods are not sequence-specific.
b.	More difficult primer design. Primer design requirements constrain target sites selection and it can limit the procedure resolution of specificity.
c.	Difficult to run multi-plex LAMP.
d.	LAMP products are not suitable for down stream.

Loop Mediated Isothermal Amplification (LAMP) is a technique similar in purpose to the older polymerase chain reaction used for the rapid amplification of nucleic acid. Requirements of LAMP are primer, enzyme and template preparation (Dhama et al., 2014). Different versions of LAMP are micro LAMP, LAMP combined with lateral flow assay (LFA), Lyophilized LAMP, Electeric LAMP (eLAMP), and Multiplex LAMP (mLAMP) (Dhama et al., 2014). It is a powerful innovative gene amplification technique emerging as a simple rapid diagnostic tool for early detection and identification of microbial diseases. LAMP does not need expensive thermocylers, as are required for PCR, because LAMP is an isothermal process. LAMP is also able to efficiently amplify RNA sequences through combination with reverse transcription. It also turns out that LAMP is more resistant than PCR to inhibitors present in complex samples such as blood. LAMP is a low-cost, rapid, highly selective and sensitive process which allows scientists to carry out DNA amplification in different settings and for different purposes (Abdullahi et al., 2015). LAMP is applicable for detection, point-of-care or field-based detection, limited resource settings, small test menu, and rapid testing, but it is inappropriate for large test menu and detection of un-sequenced targets. LAMP-based molecular assays are less versatile than PCR assays, multiplexing is difficult, and reaction volumes may be larger than in PCR, and more consumables may be required. The most important disadvantages of LAMP are shown in Table 10.

Chapter 13

Recombinase Polymerase Amplification (RPA)

Recombinase polymerase amplification (RPA) is a new isothermal method to amplify the DNA as well as RPA. RPA combines the advantages of isothermal PCR with simplicity and rapid amplification (Moody et al., 2016). It was first reported in 2006 and has been shown to improve the detection of genetically modified organisms (GMOs) (Liu et al., 2020). RPA is becoming an important technique for the rapid, sensitive, and cost-effective detection of plant viruses (Babu et al., 2018; Zhai et al., 2019). Application of RPA in cancer research is aimed at identifying the genetic defect and preventing the genetic disorder. Recombinase polymerase amplification (RPA) technique allows rapid and simple isothermal amplification of molecular targets (Glais and Jacquot, 2015). RPA assays in general demonstrated a lower tendency for false results in black control solutions of necrotic ring spot and summer patch relative to LAMP (Karakkat et al., 2018). This system is also useful for better diagnosis of pathogens by increasing the capture efficiency of the pathogen in large samples (Dao et al., 2018). Gaige et al., (2018) developed a recombinase polymerase amplification assay coupled with a lateral flow device for the specific and sensitive detection from inoculated plants using a crude DNA extraction method of *Verticillium* alfalfae. Yang et al., (2020) reported that application of the isothermal recombinase polymerase amplification-lateral flow strip (RPA-LFS) assay provided a rapid, accurate, and convenient *Vibrio parahaemolyticus* detection method which is suitable for on-site detection in resource-limited conditions compared to bioassay and quantitative PCR. Chi et al., (2020) reported that a visual detection method of LFD-RPA assay is suitable for onsite surveys and routine diagnostics and molecular identification of *Meloidogyne javanica.* The real-time RPA detection method was successfully used to amplify and detect DNA from samples of four major genetically modified crops, namely maize, rice, cotton, and soybean (Xu et al., 2014). RPA assay was also developed for detection of the toxic marine microalgae *Karlodinium veneficum* and *Karlodinium armiger* (Toldra et al., 2018). The RPA assay also exhibited a high specificity for MiCV and is simple, fast, cost effective and as sensitive as the nested PCR (Ge et al., 2018). RPA-LFD assay is highly sensitive and specific with common saffron adulterants (Zhao et al., 2019). Higgins et al., (2018) reported duplex RPA assays for the detection of bacterial meningitis pathogens: *S. pneumoniae*, *N. meningitidis*, and *H. influenzae*. Liu et al., (2021) used recombinase polymerase amplification with CRISPR-Cas12a for nucleic acid detection in the food safety field. RPA assays could be used on-site as a rapid and mobile detection system to determine contamination of products (Kissenkotter et al., 2020).

Table 11. Various recombinase amplification market on the basis of by product type, technology type, application type and user type

Type	
Product type	
a. Instrument	Microfluidic droplet generator
	Mixing incubator
	Micro ball dispenser
	Nucleic acid detection device
	Isothermal device
b. Reagents and chemicals	
c. Kits	
Technology type	
a. Microfluidic digital droplet recombinase polymerase amplification	
b. Lateral flow strip detection	
c. A real time fluorescence assay	
d. Quantitative polymerase chain reaction	
e. Gel electrophoresis	
f. Fluocculation assay	
g. ELISA	
h. Chemiluminescent detection	
i. Flow-based microarrays	
Application type	
a. Cancer research	
b. Veterinary science	
c. Clinical diagnostic	
d. Forensic testing	
e. Pathogen detection	
f. Drug discovery	
g. Biodefense	
h. Food contamination tests	
User type	
a. Diagnostic laboratories	
b. Academic institutes and research institutes	
c. Clinical research organizations	
d. Forensic laboratories	

Table 12. Advantages and disadvantages of RPA

Advantages	Disadvantages
1. Short reaction time (about 20 minutes).	1. Non-specific binding of recombinase enzyme may lead to false positive.
2. Feasibility and the ability to conduct the assay without the need of highly expensive settings which make it suitable for point of care use and in resource poor setting.	2. Instant amplification after mixing the reagents means loss of early data.
3. The flexibility of the test to accommodate varied targets as many kits were developed for different target detection.	3. The false amplification of negative control samples. Negative controls are other targets similar in feature to the original target.

Table 13. The differences between polymerase chain reaction (PCR) and recombinase polymerase amplification (RPA) in features (Abukhalid and Pastey, 2017)

Feature/Technology	Polymerase chain reaction (PCR)	Recombinase Polymerase Amplification (RPA)
Principle	Thermal nucleic acid amplification technique, consisting of 3 steps: denaturation, annealing and elongation at different temperatures.	Isothermal nucleic acid amplification technique, consist of 3 enzymes: recombinase, single strand binding protein (SSB) and strand displacing DNA polymerase.
Specificity and Sensitivity	Specificity/low, the amplicon may lose its specificity from over-amplification (above 40 cycles). Sensitivity/high, because the reaction take place under highly controlled parameters.	Specificity/high, because the amplification is based on specific binding site with relatively long primers. Sensitivity/low, because of the non-specific binding with non-homologous sequence identity of the primers and probe with the closely related negative control targets.
Convenience	Needs many steps with costly equipment.	Rapid procedures can be done with cheap resources.
Detection formats	Fluorescence	Fluorescence and Lateral flow.

It is also an accurate tool for point-of-care testing of *Norovirus*. Various recombinase amplifications marketed on the basis of byproduct type, technology type, application type and user type are shown in Table 11. Advantages and disadvantages of RPA are presented in Table 12. The differences between polymerase chain reaction (PCR) and recombinase polymerase amplification (RPA) in features are shown in Table 13.

Table 14. The mechanisms and action of RPA for various pathogens and diseases

Diseases and pathogens	**Mechanism**	**Reference**
Campylobacter jejuni	a. Real-time RPA was shown to be a simple, rapid and reliable method for *Campylobacter jejuni* detection.	Geng et al., (2019)
Mycobacterium tuberculosis	a. The LF-RPA assay can detect as low as 25 fg of *M. tuberculosis* H37Rv genomic DNA, which makes it a rapid, simple and robust method. b. Automated sample-to-answer detection of drug-resistant *M. tuberculosis* by RPA on lab-on-a-disc in 15 min.	Ma et al., (2017) Law et al., (2018)
Actinobacillus pleuropneumoniae	a. A real-time RPA assay was shown to be simple, rapid and reliable in *A. pleuropneumoniae* detection.	Li et al., (2019)
Caprine arthritis-encephalitis (CAE)	a. The RPA-LFD had significantly higher CAEV-positive rate than ELISA assay. This assay provides a specific and sensitive platform for detecting CAEV proviral DNA in goat.	Tu et al., (2017)
Penaeus stylirostris densovirus (PstDV)	a. RPA-based assay was developed for primary detection of PstDV; RPA assay is 10 fold more sensitive than a non-nested PCR which is suitable for screening in both laboratory and field application.	Jaroenram and Owens (2014)
Porcine parvovirus (PPV)	a. RPA assay provides a rapid, sensitive and specific alternative for PPV detection when compared to real-time (qPCR). b. Real-time RPA was shown to be a simple, rapid and reliable method for PPV detection.	Yang et al., (2016) Wang et al., (2017)
Porcine circovirus 2 (PCV-2)	a. RPA assay is a simple, rapid and cost-effective method for PCV-2 detection. It showed the same sensitivity as rtPCR but was 10 times more sensitive than conventional PCR. b. The novel CPV-2 LFS RPA assay is an attractive and promising tool for rapid and convenient diagnosis of CPV diseases. Moreover assay was incubated successfully in a closed fist using body heat.	Wang et al., (2016) Liu et al., (2018)
Porcine circoviurs 3 (PCV-3)	a. Real-time RPA was shown to be a simple, rapid and reliable method for PCV-3 detection.	Wang et al., (2017)
Porcine epidemic diarrhea virus (PEDV)	a. The developed RT-RPA assay provides a useful alternative tool for simple, rapid and reliable detection of PEDV in resource-limited diagnostic laboratories and on-site facilities.	Wang et al., (2018)
Canine distemper virus (CDV)	a. The novel CDV LFS RT-RPA assay provides an attractive and promising tool for rapid and reliable detection of CDV.	Wang et al., (2018)

Diseases and pathogens	Mechanism	Reference
Canine parvovirus 2 (CPV-2)	a. The novel CPV-2 LFS RPA assay is an attractive and promising too for rapid and convenient diagnosis of CPV disease.	Liu et al., (2018)
Pseudorabies virus (PRV)	a. The RPA assay provides a rapid, sensitive and specific alternative for detection of PRV.	Yang et al., (2017)
Respiraotry syncytial virus (RSV)	a. A RT-RPA assay was established for the detection of RSV which was faster than RT-qPCR. b. The RT-RPA-LFD assay could simultaneously detect RSV subtype A and B with the same detection limit.	Xi et al., (2019) Xu et al., (2020)
Rice black-streaked dwarf virus (RBSDV)	a. The RBSDV RT-RPA assay developed as a successful tool for quick diagnosis of RBSDV-infected rice plants.	Zhao et al., (2019)
Verticillum dahliae	a. An RPA-LFD assay was developed for the rapid and visual detection of *V. dahliae* within 25 min. b. The detection limit of the RPA-LFD assay was 103 fg fungal genomic DNA and was equal to that of conventional PCR. c. The RPA-LFD assay detected *V. dahliae* from samples, and its sensitivity was 10 times higher than conventional PCR.	Ju et al., (2020)
Yellow mosaic virus (ZYMV)	a. RPA was coupled with enzyme-assisted signal amplification (EASA) by circularizing one strand of RPA product. A cyclic ssDNA was obtained using RPA product, T4 DNA ligase and T5 exonuclease.	Wang et al., (2020)
Mycoplasma hyopneumoniae	a. The developed RPA assays are suitable for rapid and reliable detection of *M. hyopneumoniae* in diagnostic laboratory and at point-of-need facility.	Liu et al., (2019)
Chlamydia trachomatis	a. RPA assay uses recombinase polymerase amplification and has a minimum detection limit of 5 to 12 pathogens per test.	Krolov et al., (2014)
Streptococcus pyogenes (GAS)	a. Propidium monoazie (PMA)-RPA assay has been developed for its detection.	Chen et al., (2018)
Streptococcus agalactiae (GBS)	a. Propidium monoazie (PMA)-RPA has been developed for its detection.	Chen et al., (2018) Hu et al., (2019)
Dengue virus (DENV)	a. RT-RPA assay constituents a suitable accurate, sensitive and rapid assay for dengue fever diagnosis during the first 5 days of infection. b. A RT-RPA-LFD assay was developed for the detection of DENV which was faster than RT-qPCR.	El Wahed et al., (2014) Xi et al., (2019)
Bovine leukemia virus (BLV)	a. RPA-LFD method is appropriate for detecting BLV nucleic acid at a lower limit. It can serve as an alternative tool to ELISA for the preliminary screening of BLV for its simplicity and portability.	Tu et al., (2018)

Table 14. (Continued)

Diseases and pathogens	Mechanism	Reference
Bovine coronavirus (BCoV)	a. RPA assay was developed for the detection of bovine coronavirus, and the assay was rapid (10-20 min), with analytical sensitivity of 19 RNA molecules and specific. The combination of this assay with a new portable fluorescence reader is a new step toward point-of-care nucleic acid detection.	Amer et al., (2013)
Bovine parainfluenza virus type 3 (BPIV3)	a. A LFD RT-RPA assay was developed for detection of BPIV3. Compared to qPCR, the LFD RT-RPA assay showed a clinical sensitivity of 94.74% and a clinical specificity of 96.05%.	Zhao et al., (2018)
Goose parvovirus (GPV)	a. The GPV-RPA-VF (Vertical flow) assay was accurate, sensitive and specific for detection of GPV and N-GPV. The assay yielded the same results as qPCR on detecting virus in field blood samples.	Liu et al., (2019)
Avian Influenza (H5N1)	a. RT-RPA assay was developed for detection of H5N1 virus in clinical samples.	Ahmed et al., (2020)
Influenza A virus (subtype H1 and H3)	a. The sensitivity of RT-RPA-LFD assay is lower than that of real-time RT-PCR, comparable or better than that of conventional RT-PCR.	Sun et al., (2018)
Plasmodium knowlesi	a. RPA's combination with SYBR Green I is fast and easy to perform which is suitable for use in resource-limited settings.	Lai and Lau (2020)
Staphylococcus aureus	a. RPA-PFS (Polymer flocculation sedimentation) was highly specific for *S. aureus* and the results can be directly observed by the naked eye without any equipment.	Hu et al., (2020)
Toxoplasma gondii	a. B1-LF-RPA was a promising method as a molecular detection tool for *T. gondii*, and its sensitivity was 10 times higher than that of nest PCR.	Wu et al., (2017)
Grass carp (*Ctenopharyngodon idella*) reovirus (GCRV)	a. The real-time RT-RPA assay was developed for the detection of GCRV genotype III, and the assay is useful for resource-limited diagnostic laboratories.	Wang et al., (2020)
Legionella spp.	a. In-house RPA primer design for the detection of *Legionella* spp. and *L. pneumophila*.	Kober et al., (2018)
Cyprinid herpesvirus 3 (CyHV-3)	a. The RPA assay and lateral flow device provide for the rapid, sensitive and specific amplification of CyHV-3.	Prescott et al., (2016)
Atypical pneumonia	a. RPA is suggested for near patient and field testing with a rather simple routine and the possibility for a read out with the naked eye.	Kersting et al., (2018)
Enterocytozoon hepatopenaei (EHP)	a. The sensitivity of EHP-RPA was higher than PCR but lower than real-time PCR.	Zhou et al., (2020)

Diseases and pathogens	Mechanism	Reference
Shrimp hemocyte iridescent virus (SHIV)	a. The RPA assay provides a rapid, accurate, sensitive, affordable and specific alternative for detection of SHIV.	Chen et al., (2020)
Salmonella	a. The real-time RPA assay was considerable faster than qPCR and exhibited no losses in detection sensitivity and specificity.	Hu et al., (2019) Hong et al., (2020)
Apple stem pitting virus (ASPV)	a. The RT-RPA assay could detect ASPV in a reaction time of only 1 min. It showed high sensitivity and specificity for detecting ASPV in pear samples.	Kim et al., (2019)
Potato virus Y and X	a. The RPA assay efficiently detects viral RNA in low viral titer samples, including the peridermal tissues of potato tubers. b. Recombinase polymerase amplification-lateral flow assay for potato virus X was developed, and detection limit was 0.14 ng potato virus X per g potato leaves.	Babujee et al., (2019) Ivanov et al., (2020) Wang et al., (2020)
Potato mop-top virus (PMTV)	a. The developed RPA assay may provide a useful alternative tool for the rapid, simple and reliable detection of Spongospora subterranean f. sp. subterranea (Sss) and PMTV in diagnostic laboratories and in-field testing.	DeShields et al., (2019)
Peach latent mosaic viroid (PLMVD)	a. RT-RPA assay can detect PLMVD in only 5 minutes. It showed high sensitivity and specificity for detecting PLMVD	Lee et al., (2020)
Plum pox virus (PPV)	a. Isothermal AmplifyRP® using reverse transcription-recombinase polymerase amplification was reported as an innovative technique to detect rapidly plant viruses affecting perennial crops.	Zhang et al., (2014)
Cucumer mosaic virus (CMV)	a. A highly sensitive fluorescence-based real-time RT-exo-RPA assay has been developed for the rapid detection of Cucumer mosaic virus.	Srivastava et al., (2019)
Cucumer green mottle mosaic virus (CGMMV)	a. RPA method was more sensitive compared with the regular RT-PCR for CGMMV detection in water melon in resource-limited laboratories or on-site facilities. b. CGMMV RT-RPA was 100-fold more sensitive than the normal RT-PCR assay.	Jiao et al., (2019) Zeng et al., (2019)
Spring viremia of carp virus (SVCV)	a. The real-time RT-RPA assay was reported as high specific and sensitive assay for rapid detection of SVCV.	Cong et al., (2020)
Monkeypox virus (MPXV)	a. The new developed MPXV-RPA-assay is fast and can be easily utilized at low resource settings using a solar powered mobile suitcase laboratory.	Davi et al., (2019)
Theiler's murine encephalomyelitis virus (TMEV)	a. RT-RPA is more cost-effective than RT-qPCR to apply in a mobile laboratory for field detection.	Ma et al., (2018)

Table 14. (Continued)

Diseases and pathogens	Mechanism	Reference
Rose rosette virus (RRV)	a. Developed RT-RPA assays for detection or RRV were highly sensitive, detecting up to 1 fg of virus. Moreover, developed assay successfully detected RRV from leaves, stems and flower petals.	Babu et al., (2017)
Severe fever with thrombocytopenia syndrome virus (SFTSV)	a. The rapid and efficient RT-RPA assay can be a promising candidate for point-of-care detection of SFTSV.	Zhou et al., (2020)
Brucellosis	a. A rapid and sensitive Bruce-RPA was developed for detection of *Brucella*, which represents a candidate point-of-care diagnosis assay for human brucellosis. b. RPA assay may be a rapid, sensitive and specific tool for the prevention and control of Brucellosis.	Ren et al., (2016) Gumaa et al., (2019) Qin et al., (2019)
Foot-and-mouth disease virus (FMDV)	a. The developed RPA-LFD assay provides a rapid, simple, highly promising approach to be used as point-of-care diagnostics in the field.	Wang et al., (2018)
Lumpy skin disease virus (LSDV)	a. The LSDV RPA assay is a rapid and sensitive test which could be implemented in field or at quarantine stations for the identification of LSDV infected case.	Shalaby et al., (2016)
Peste des petits ruminants (PRP)	a. Conventional and real-time RT-RPA assays were developed for the detection PPRV with high sensitivity and specificity.	
Infectious spleen and kidney necrosis virus (ISKNV)	a. The RPA-LFD method achieved rapid detection of ISKNV without professional staff equipment.	Li et al., (2020)
Theileria annulata	a. The LF-RPA could be used to surveil and control of *Theileria annulata*, and its sensitivity is similar to PCR for detecting the field samples.	Yin et al., (2017) Hassan et al., (2018)
Karlodinium veneficum	a. RPA-LFD assay can be used as a rapid and sensitive method to monitor *K. veneficum*.	Fu et al., (2019)
Anaplasma phagocytophilum	a. A specific, sensitive, rapid and cost-effective RPA method was developed for the detection of *A. phagocytophilum*.	Zhao et al., (2019)
Neospora caninum	a. The LF-RPA assay can detect *N. caninum* DNA at amounts as low as 50 fg.	Tian et al., (2018)
Viruses infecting ginger	a. RT-LAMP and RT-RPA based isothermal assays were developed for quick detection of two novel viruses infecting ginger.	Naveen and Bhat (2020)
Orientia tsutsugamushi	a. The RPA-LF detection method is promising for wide-ranging use in basic medical units.	Qi et al., (2018)

Diseases and pathogens	Mechanism	Reference
Schistosoma haematobium	a. The LF-RPA assay can amplify and detect low levels of *S. haematobium* DNA.	Rosser et al., (2015)
Schistosoma mansoni	a. A LF-RPA assay has been developed for *S. mansoni*. The assay can detect 10pg of DNA and 102 copies of DNA.	Poulton and Webster (2018)
Brucella	a. Bruce-RPA was developed for detection of *Brucella*. The assay could detect as few as 3 copies of *Brucella* per reaction within 20 min.	Ren et al., (2016)
Rift Valley fever virus	a. The combination of one-step-RT-RPA and portable fluorescence reading device could be a useful tool for point of care diagnostics.	Euler et al., (2012)
HIV infection	a. RT-RPA can detect low copies of HIV-1 proviral DNA and genomic RNA. An HIV-1 assay that can detect variant target sequences in groups M and O, and the test results is available in 20 min.	Lillis et al., (2016)
Rose rosette virus (RRV)	a. The developed novel, sensitive and rapid (20 min) RT-exoRPA assay was used for its detection. The assay was highly sensitive, detecting up to 1 fg of virus.	Babu et al., (2017)
Yam mosaic virus (YMV)	a. RT-RPA test for specific detection of YMV detects as low as 14 pg/µl of viral RNA. RT-RPA was reported more suitable than RT-PCR for routine screening of YMV.	Silva et al., (2015)
Listeria monocytogenes	a. RPA methods provided reliable alternatives to conventional culture methods.	Garrido-Maestu et al., (2018)
Vibrio harveyi	a. The developed RPA assays provide a rapid, simple, sensitive and specific alternative tool for detection of *V. harveyi*.	Pang et al., (2019)
Transmissible gastroenteritis virus (TGEV)	a. A developed RT-PCR assay provides a useful alternative tool for rapid, simple and reliable detection of TGEV. The R2 value of RT-RPA and real time RT-PCR was 0.959 by linear regression analysis.	Wang et al., (2018)
Feline parvovirus (FPV)	a. RPA-LFD can detect FPV pathogen genome at 36oC-40oC for 15 min. RPA-LFD achieves immediate field detection without professional staff and sophisticated equipment and it displays higher sensitivity and lower detection costs than traditional PCR method.	Wang et al., (2019)
Marek's disease virus (MDV)	a. A real-time RPA assay was developed for rapid detection of MDV, which is highly specific and sensitive and a good alternative to PCR methods.	Zeng et al., (2019)
Flavobacterium columnare	a. A rapid on-field, isothermal RPA-LFD assay was developed to detect *F. columnare* which was more sensitive than RPA-gel electrophoresis.	Mabrok et al., (2021)
Laryngotracheitis virus	a. The real-time RPA method has shown specificity, sensitivity and reproductivity for the rapid detection of infectious laryngotracheitis virus.	Zhu et al., (2020)

RPA has been used for detection of abalone herpes-like virus (AbHV) and Red-spotted grouper nervous necrosis virus (RGNNV), which are two serious viruses that infect animal populations in aquaculture, and the detection limits are 100 viral DNA copies per reaction for both viruses and detection methods for both viruses have good specificity without false positive results (Gao et al., 2018). The mechanisms and action of RPA for various pathogens and diseases are presented in Table 14.

Chapter 14

Recombinase Aided Amplification (RAA)

The recombinase-aided amplification (RAA) assay is a new isothermal amplification technology with the advantages of rapidity, simplicity and low cost. Recombinase aided amplification (RAA) assay does not require a classical thermostable enzyme or a sophisticated thermal cycler, and enzymes used in RAA assay include single strand DNA binding protein (SSB), recombinase UvsX and DNA polymerase, and the reaction is typically completed at 39°C in 20-30 min. RAA has been successfully applied in the detection of bacterial and viral pathogens (Duan et al., 2018). It overcomes the technical difficulties posed by DNA amplification methods because it does not need thermal denaturation of the template and operates at a low and constant temperature (Uddin et al., 2016). The mechanisms and action of RAA for various pathogens and diseases are shown in Table 15.

Table 15. The mechanisms and action of RAA for various pathogens and diseases

Diseases and pathogens	**Mechanisms**	**Reference**
SARS-CoV-2	a. RT-RAA assay for SARS-CoV-2 showed the distinctive advantages for simplicity and rapidity in terms of operation and turnaround time.	Wang et al., (2020)
Respiratory syncytial virus (RSV)	a. RT-RAA correctly identified and differentiated all RSV-positive samples with 100% sensitivity and specificity compared with RT-qPCR assay. The RT-RAA detection system does not require a sophisticated laboratory setting or expensive equipment.	Chen et al., (2018) Qi et al., (2019)
Staphylococcus aureus	a. A modified propidium monoazide (PMAxx) was selected to more accurately eliminate the interference from dead cells. The assay could detect 101 CFU/mL viable cells in milk sample after 6 h enrichment.	Xie et al., (2021)
Porcine circovirus type 3 (PCV-3)	a. The PCV-3 RAA assay is a sensitive, specific and rapid method, which can be used for epidemiological studies of PCV-3 and it costs less than real-time PCR.	Li et al., (2020)
Bovine ephermeral fever virus (BEFV)	a. Isothermal recombinase polymerase amplification assay was developed to detect BEFV (LFD-RPA). The RPA combined with LFD assay probably provides an alternative for diagnosis of BEFV.	Hou et al., (2018)

Table 15. (Continued)

Diseases and pathogens	**Mechanisms**	**Reference**
Salmonella	a. RAA method for detection of *Salmonella* is sensitive, specific and rapid.	Zhang et al., (2017)
Mycoplasma pneumoniae	a. RAA assay is a fast, sensitive and specific alternative tool for the detection of *M. pneumonia*.	Xue et al., (2020)
Orf virus (ORFV)	a. The RAA assay has high sensitivity and specificity which is suitable for detection of ORFV at the grassroots level.	Wang et al., (2020)
Hepatitis B virus (HBV)	a. The RAA method is a rapid, convenient, highly sensitive and specific method to detect HBV without DNA extraction in clinical samples.	Shen et al., (2019)
Bordetella pertussis	a. RT-PCR assay has advantages of 45 min turn-around time and simple steps of DNA purification and it is a useful diagnostic tool for its detection.	Zhang et al., (2019)
Human adenovirus (HAdV)	a. Duplex RAA assay effectively reduces the rate of false negative results and may be valuable for detection of HAdV 3 and HAdV 7 in clinical laboratories.	Wang et al., (2019)
Dengue virus (DENV)	a. RT-RAA-LFD assay with high specificity and sensitivity is visual, rapid and reliable for DENV detection.	Xion et al., (2020)

Conclusion

Different isothermal amplification methods are the signal amplification assays, the probe amplification assays, and the target amplification assays. Molecular techniques used for recognition of quinolone resistance consist of the use of various techniques such as polymerase chain reaction fragment length polymorphism, PCR, single-strand conformation polymorphism, nucleotide-sequencing analysis and multiplex allele-specific polymerase chain reaction. Main nucleic acid testing techniques are amplified nucleic acid techniques, microarrays, and non-amplified acid techniques. Non-amplified nucleic acid techniques consist of DNA labeled probes, and RNA labeled probes. Molecular methods have considerable benefits for the programmatic management of drug resistant. The PCR-based methods have high sensitivity, specificity, but several molecular tests which employ non-PCR-based methods are developed for rapid detection of RNA such as isothermal nucleic acid amplification like loop mediated isothermal amplification and nucleic acid sequence-based amplification. The most notable methods which can be used to detect the pathogens are biochemical assays, immunological assays and polymerase chain reaction (PCR)-based testing of bacterial nucleic acids. The reliability and sensitivity of PCR assay depend on DNA quality. PCR methods are also powerful techniques which revolutionized molecular biology by offering applications in the diagnosis of microbial infections and genetic diseases, as well as in detection of pathogens in food. The real-time PCR method can be more specific and involves complex processing steps and requires prior sequence data of the specific target gene. Loop-mediated isothermal amplification (LAMP) is a powerful and specific DNA-based detection method which can be used on-site. LAMP methods can be more specific than qPCR and immunoassays. Loop-mediated isothermal amplification can be used for detection of both DNA and RNA viruses, and apply for diagnosis of various important emerging and re-emerging diseases. LAMP rapidly amplifies nucleic acids with high specificity and sensitivity under isothermal conditions. LAMP technology has been widely used for the detection of human pathogenic bacteria, crop pests, pathogenic organisms and components in meat products. The LAMP assay can be used in the field of molecular diagnosis of cancer, identification of genetically modified organisms, detection of food adulteration, eutrophication, food allergens, pesticides, identification of medicinal plants, drug resistance and DNA methylation studies. The LAMP assay can be used for rapid detection of SARS-CoV, MERS-CoV, SARS-CoV-2, influenza, lymphocystis disease virus, swine acute diarrhea syndrome coronavirus, swine vesicular disease virus, classical swine fever virus, infectious bursal disease virus, Marek's disease virus, human papillomaviruses, infectious bronchitis virus, Newcastle disease virus, sacbrood virus, beak and feather disease virus, foot-and-mouth disease virus, bovine herpesvirus-1, milk vetch dwarf virus and etc. PCR is a very sensitive technique which allows rapid amplification of a specific segment of DNA; PCR makes billions of copies of a specific DNA fragment or gene, which allows detection and identification of gene sequences using visual techniques based on size and charge, and modified versions of PCR have allowed quantitative measurements of gene expression with techniques called real-time PCR. The most important limitations of PCR method consiss of the DNA polymerase used in the PCR reaction is prone to errors and can lead to mutations in the fragment generated, the specificity of the generated PCR product may be altered by nonspecific binding of the primers to other similar sequences on the template DNA, and to design primers to generate a PCR product, some prior sequence information is usually necessary. Contamination or nonspecific priming can lead to false-positive results, and the most concern is that PCR detects nucleic acids whether or not they come from viable cells. LAMO is much more sensitive and specific when compared to PCR or detection of viral diseases. Recombinase Polymerase Amplification is a relatively new isothermal methodology for amplifying DNA. It has developed as an alternative to PCR assay which can amplify nucleic acids at 37°C-39°C within 20 min. PCR relies on repeated heating and cooling cycles to denature and amplify DNA fragments, RPA is performed at a single moderate temperature and uses enzymatic activity to drive amplification. Moreover, RPA is mostly common in field-based monitoring of pathogens. Recombinase aided amplification (RAA) assay has been successfully applied in the detection of bacterial and viral pathogens and overcomes the technical difficulties posed by DNA amplification methods because it does not need thermal denaturation of the template and operates at a low and constant temperature.

References

Abou El-Khier, N. T., El Sayed Zaki, M. (2020). Molecular detection and frequency of fluoroquinolone-resistant Escherichia coli by multiplex allele specific polymerase chain reaction (MAS-PCR). *Egypt J Basic Appl Sci. 7*(1), 1-7.

Adachi, D., Johnson, G., Draker, R., Ayers, M., Mazzulli, T., Talbot, P. J., Tellier, R., (2004). Comprehensive detection and identification of human coronaviruses, including the SARS-associated coronavirus, with a single RT-PCR assay. *J Virol Methods. 122*(1), 29-36.

Afzal, A. (2020). Molecular diagnostic technologies for COVID-19: Limitations and challenges. *J Adv Res*. http://doi.org/10.1016/j.jare.2020.08.002.

Ahmed, B. M., Amer, H. A., Kissenkoetter, J., El-Wahed, A. A., Bayoumi, M. M., Bohlken-Fascher, S., Elgamal, M. A., Yehia, N., Yousif, A. A., Shalaby, M. A. (2020). Evaluating two approaches for using positive control in standardizing the avian influenza H5 reverse transcription recombinase polymerase amplification assay. *Mol Cell probe. 50*, 101511.

Akashi, Y., Suzuki, H., Ueda, A., Hirose, Y., Hayashi, D., Imai, H., Ishikawa, H. (2019). Analytical and clinical evaluation of a point-of-care molecular diagnostic system and its influenza A/B assay for rapid molecular detection of the influenza virus. *J Infect Chemother. 25*, 578-583.

Ali, Z., Aman, R., Mahas, A., Rao, G. S., Tehseen, M., Marsic, T., Salunke, R., Subudhi, A. K., Hala, S. M., Hamdan, S. M., Pain, A., Alofi, F. S., Alsomali, A., Hashem, A.M., Khogeer, A., Almontashiri, N. A. M., Abedalthagafi, M., Hassan, N., Mahfouz, M. M. (2020). iSCAN: An RT-LAMP-coupled CRISPR-Cas12 module for rapid, sensitive detection of SARS-CoV-2. *Virus Res. 288*, 198129.

Allawi, H. T., Dahlberg, J. E., Olson, S., Lund, E., Olson, M., Ma, W. P., Takova, T., Neri, B. P., Lyamichev, V. I. (2004). Quantitation of microRNAs using a modified invader assay. *RNA. 10*(7), 1153-1161.

Alnefaie, A., Albogami, S. (2020). Current approaches used in treating COVID-19 from a molecular mechanisms and immune response perspective. *Saudi Pharm J.* doi: 10.1016/j.jsps.2020.08.024.

Alvarez-Diaz, D. A., Franco-Munoz, C., Laiton-Donato, K., Usme-Ciro, J. A., Franco-Sierra, N., Florez-Sanchez, A. C., Gomez-Rangel, S., Rodriguez-Calderon, L. D., Barbosa-Ramirez, J., Ospitia-Baez, E., Walteros, D. M., Ospina-Martinez, M. L., Mercado-Reyes, M. (2020). Molecular analysis of several in-house rRT-PCR protocols for SARS-CoV-2 detection in the context of genetic variability of the virus in Colombia. *Infect Genet Evol. 84*, 104390.

Amagliani, G., Parlani, M. L., Brandi, G., Sebastianelli, G., Stocchi, V., Schiavano, G. F. (2012). Molecular detection of Pseudomonas aeruginosa in recreational water. *Int J Environ Health Res. 22*(1), 60-70.

Aman, R., Mahas, A., Mahfouz, M. (2020). Nucleic acid detection using CRISPR/cas biosensing technologies. *ACS Synth Biol. 9*, 1226-1233.

An, L., Tang, W., Ranalli, T. A., Kim, H. J., Wytiaz, J., Kong, H. (2005). Characterization of thermostable UvrD helicase and its participation in helicase-dependent amplification. *J Biol Chem. 280*(32), 28952-28958.

Anker, J. N., Hall, W. P., Lyandres, O., Shah, N. C., Zhao, J., Van Duyne, R. P. (2008). Biosensing with plasmonic nanosensors. *Nat Mater. 7*, 442-453.

Attwood, L. O., Francis, M. J., Hamblin, J., Korman, T. M., Druce, J., Graham, M. (2020). Clinical evaluation of AusDiagnostics SARS-CoV-2 multiplex tandem PCR assay. *J Clin Virol. 128*, 104448.

Baek, Y. H., Um, J., Antigua, K. J. C., Park, J. H., Kim, Y., Oh, S., Kim, Y. I., Choi, W. S., Kim, S. G., Jeong, J. H., Chin, B. S., Dawn, H., Nicolas, H. D. G., Ahn, J. Y., Shin, K. S., Choi, Y. K., Park, J. S., Song, M.-S. (2020). Development of a reverse transcription-loop-mediated isothermal amplification as a rapid early-detection method for novel SARS-CoV-2. *Emerg Microbes Infect. 9*(1), 998-1007.

Ball, C., Felice, V., Ding, Y., Forrester, A., Catelli, E., Ganapathy, K. (2020). Influences of swab types and storage temperatures on isolation and molecular detection of Mycoplasma gallisepticum and Mycoplasma synoviae. *Avian Pathol. 49*(1), 106-110.

Barken, K. B., Haagensen, J. A., Tolker-Nielsen, T. (2007). Advances in nucleic acid-based diagnostics of bacterial infections. *Clin Chim Acta. 384*, 1-11.

Barletta, J., Bartolome, A. (2007). Immuno-polymerase chain reaction as a unique molecular tool for detection of infectious agents. *Expert Opin Med Diagn. 1*(2), 267-288.

Barza, R., Patel, P., Sabatini, L., Singh, K. (2020). Use of a simplified sample processing step without RNA extraction for direct SARS-CoV-2 RT-PCR detection. *Journal of Clinical Virology. 132*, 104587.

Bhadra, S., Jiang, Y. S., Kumar, M. R., et al., (2015). Real-time sequence-validated loop-mediated isothermal amplification assays for detection of Middle East respiratory syndrome coronavirus (MERS-CoV). *PLOS ONE. 10*(4), e0123126.

Bourhis, Y., Gottwald, T. R., Lopez-Ruiz, F. J., Patarapuwadol, S., van den Bosch, F. (2019). Sampling for disease absence-deriving informed monitoring from epidemic traits. *J Theor Biol. 461*, 8-16.

Boutin, C. A., Grandjean-Lapierre, S., Gagnon, S., Labbe, A. C., Charest, H., Roger, M., Coutlee, F. (2020). Comparison of SARS-CoV-2 detection from combined nasopharyngeal/oropharyngeal swab samples by a laboratory-developed real-time RT-PCR test and the Roche SARS-CoV-2 assay on a cobas 8800 instrument. *J Clin Virol. 132*, 104615.

Braga, M., Costa, F. N., Gomes, D. R. M., Zavier, D. R., Andre, M. R., Goncalves, L. R., Freschi, C. R., Machado, R. Z. (2017). Genetic diversity of piroplasmids species in equids from island of Sao Luis, northeastern Brazil. *Rev Bras Parasitol Vet. 26*, 331-339.

Bremer, J., Nowicki, M., Beckner, S., Brambilla, D., Cronin, M., Herman, S., Kovacs, A., Reichelderfer, P. (2000). Comparison of two amplification technologies for detection and quantitation of human immunodeficiency virus type 1 RNA in the female genital tract. Division of AIDS treatment research initiative 009 study team. *J Clin Microbiol. 38*(7), 2665-2669.

Brossier, F., Sougakoff, W., Aubry, A., Bernard, C., Cambau, E., Jarlier, V., Mougari, F., Raskine, L., Robert, J., Veziris, N. (2017). Molecular detection methods of resistance to antituberculosis drugs in Mycobacterium tuberculosis. *Med Mal Infect. 47*, 340-348.

Broughton, J. P., Deng, X., Yu, G., Fasching, C. L., Servellita, V., Singh, J., Miao, X., Streithorst, J. A., Granados, A., Sotomayor-Gonzalez, A., et al., (2020). CRISPR-Cas12-based detection of SARS-CoV-2. *Nat Biotechnol. 38*, 870-874.

Bordi, L., Piralla, A., Lalle, E., Giardina, F., Colavita, F., Tallarita, M., Sberna, G., Novazzi, F., Meschi, S., Castilletti, C., Brisci, A., Minnucci, G., Tettamanzi, V., Baldanti, F., Capobianchi, M.,R. (2020). Rapid and sensitive detection of SARS-CoV-2 RNA using Simplexa^{TM} COVID-19 direct assay. *J Clin Virol. 128*, 104416.

Budiarto, B. R., Pohan, P. U., Desriani. (2019). Nucleic acid amplification-based HER2^{I655V} molecular detection for breast cancer. *J Oncol Sci. 5*(1): 31-41.

Bwanga, F., Hoffner, S., Haile, M., Joloba, M. L. (2009). Direct susceptibility testing for multi drug resistant tuberculosis: a meta-analysis. *BMC Infect Dis. 9*, 67.

Cao, Y. W. C., Jin, R. C., Mirkin, C. A. (2002). Nanoparticles with Raman spectroscopic fingerprints for DNA and RNA detection. *Science. 297*, 1536-1540.

Cao, Y., Feng, T., Xu, J., Xue, C. (2019). Recent advances of molecularly imprinted polymer-based sensors in the detection of food safety hazard factors. *Biosens Bioelectron. 141*, 111447.

Chen, W., Li, S., Shao, B., Zheng, T., Jiang, S., Huang, X., Cai, K., Zhang, Z. (2004). Preliminary study on detecting the SARS-CoV specific target cDNA fragments by multiplex PCR. *Genom Proteom Bioing. 2*(1), 55-58.

Chen, C., Li, X. N., Li, C. Z., Zhao, L., Duan, S. X., Yan, T. F., Feng, Z. S., Ma, X. J. (2018). Use of a rapid reverse-transcription recombinase aided amplification assay for respiratory syncytial virus detection. *Diagn Microbiol Infect Dis. 90*(2), 90-95.

Cho, E. J., Yang, L., Levy, M., Ellington, A. D. (2005). Using a deoxyribozyme ligase and rolling circle amplification to detect a non-nucleic acid analyte. *ATP J Am Chem. Soc. 127*(7), 2022-2023.

Cholleti, H., Berg, M., Hayer, J., Blomstrom, A.-L. (2018). Vector-borne viruses and their detection by viral metagenomics. *Infect Ecol Epidemiol. 8*(1), 1553465.

Christaki, E. (2015). New technologies in predicting, preventing and controlling emerging infectious diseases. *Virulence. 6*(6), 558-565.

Cobo, F. (2012). Application of molecular diagnostic techniques for viral testing. *Open Virol J. 6*, 104-113.

Corman, V. M., Landt, O., Kaiser, M., et al., (2020). Detection of 2019 novel coronavirus (2019-nCoV) by real-time RT-PCR. *Euro Surveill. 25*, 23-30.

Cordes, A. K., Heim, A. (2020). Rapid random access detection of the novel SARS-coronavirus-2 (SARS-CoV-2, previously 2019-nCoV) usig an open access protocol for the Panther Fusion. *J Clin Virol. 125*, 104305.

Cunniffe, N. J., Cobb, R. C., Meentemeyer, R. K., Rizzo, D. M., Gilligan, C. A. (2016). Modeling when, where and how to manage a forest epidemic, motivated by sudden oak death in California. *Proc Nat Acad Sci.* 201602153.

Dean, F. B., Nelson, J. R., Giesler, T. L., Lasken, R. S. (2001). Rapid amplification of plasmid and phage DNA using Phi 29 DNA polymerase and multiply-primed rolling circle amplification. *Genome Res. 11*(6), 1095-1099.

Deborah, J. E., Emesto, K., Martin, J. W., et al., (2002). Detection gyrA mutations in quinolone-resistant Salmonella enteric by denaturing high-performance liquid chromatography. *J Clin Microbiol. 40*, 4121-4125.

Decousser, J. W., Poirel, L., Nordmann, P. (2017). Recent advances in biochemical and molecular diagnostics for the rapid detection of antibiotic-resistant Enterobacteriaceae: a focus on β-lactam resistance. *Expert Rev Mol Diagn. 17*(4), 327-350.

Demidov, V. V. (2002). Rolling-circle amplification DNA diagnostics: the power of simplicity. *Expert Rev Mol Diagn. 2*(6), 542-548.

Deng, R., Zhang, K., Li, J. (2017). Isothermal application for MicroRNA detection: from the test tube to the cell. *Acc Chem Res. 50*(4), 1059-1068.

Diggle, M. A., Clarke, S. C. (2006). Molecular methods for the detection and characterization of Neisseria meningitidis. *Expert Rev Mol Diagn. 6*(1), 79-87.

Dong, L., Zhou, J., Niu, C., Wang, Q., Pan, Y., Sheng, S., Wang, X., Zhang, Y., Yang, J., Liu, M., et al., (2020). Highly accurate and sensitive diagnostic detection of SARS-CoV-2 by digital PCR. *MedRxiv*. doi: 10.1101/2020.03.14.20036129.

Du, X., Zhou, J. (2018). Application of biosensors to detection of epidemic diseases in animals. *Res Vet Sci. 118*, 444-448.

Duffy, K. J., Littrell, J., Locke, A., Sherman, S. L., Olivier, M. (2008). A novel procedure for genotyping of single nucleotide polymorphisms in trisomy with genomic DNA and the invader assay. *Nucleic Acids Res. 36*(22), e145.

Engstrom, A. (2016). Fighting an old disease with modern tools: characteristics and molecular detection methods of drug-resistant Mycobacterium tuberculosis. *Infect Dis. 48*(1), 1-17.

Enosawa, M., Kageyama, S., Sawai, K., Watanabe, K., Notomi, T., Onoe, S., Mori, Y., Yokomizo, Y. (2003). Use of loop-mediated isothermal amplification of the IS900 sequence for rapid detection of cultured *Mycobacterium avium subsp. Paratuberc J Clin Microbiol. 41*(9), 4359-4365.

Fenollar, F., Raoult, D. (2004). Molecular genetic methods for the diagnosis of fastidious microorganisms. *Ampis. 112*, 785-807.

Ferreira, J. D. S., Carvalho, F. M. D., Pessolani, M. C. V., Antunes, J. M. A. D. P., Oliveira, I. V. P. D. M., Moura, G. H. F., Truman, R. W., Pena, M. T., Sharma, R., Duthie, M. S., Guimaraes, R. J. D. P. S., Fontes, A. N. B., NoelSuffys, P., McIntosh, D. (2020). Serological and molecular detection of infection with Mycobacterium leprae in Brazilian six banded armadillos (Euphractus sexcinctus). *Comp Immunol, Microbiol Infect Dis. 68*, 101397.

Gan, S. D., Patel, K. R. (2013). Enzyme immunoassay and enzyme-linked immunosorbent assay. *J Investing Dermatol. 133*, 1-3.

Gao, W., Li, X., Zeng, L., Peng, T. (2008). Rapid isothermal detection assay: a probe amplification method for the detection of nucleic acids. *Diagn Microbiol Infect Dis. 60*(2), 133-141.

Gilchrist, S., Kinchesh, P., Zarghami, M., Khrapitchev, A. A., Sibson, N. R., Kersemans, V., Smart, S. C. (2020). Improved detection of molecularly targeted iron oxide particles in mouse brain using B_0 field stabilized high resolution MRI. *Magn Reson Imaging. 57*, 101-108.

Gill, P., Ramezani, R., Amiri, M. V., Ghaemi, A., Hashempour, T., Eshraghi, N., Ghalami, M., Tehrani, H. A. (2006). Enzyme-linked immunosorbent assay of nucleic acid sequence-based amplification for molecular detection of M. Tuberculosis. *Bioche Biophys Res Commun. 347*(4), 1151-1157.

Gill, P., Amini, M., Ghaemi, A., Shokouhizadeh, L., Abdul-Tehrani, A., Karami, A., Gilak, A. (2007). Detection of Helicobacter pylori by enzyme-linked immunosorbent assay of thermophilic helicase-dependent isothermal DNA amplification. *Diagn Microbiol Infect Dis. 59*(3), 243-249.

Guichon, A., Chiparelli, H., Martinez, A., Rodriguez, C., Trento, A., Russia, J. C., Carballal, G. (2004). Evaluation of a new NASBA assay for the qualitative detection of hepatitis C virus based on the NucliSens Basic Kit reagents. *J Clin Virol. 29*(2), 84-91.

Haldavnekar, R., Venkatakrishnan, K., Tan, B. (2020). Next generation SERS-atomic scale platform for molecular level detection. *Appl Mater Today. 18*, 100529.

Hall, M. J., Wharam, S. D., Weston, A., Cardy, D. L., Wilson, W. H. (2002). Use of signal mediated amplification of RNA technology (SMART) to detect marine cyanophage DNA. *Biotechniques. 32*(3), 604-6, 608-11.

Hirotsu, Y., Mochizuki, H., Omata, M. (2020). Double-quencher probes improve detection sensitivity toward severe acute respiratory syndrome coronavirus 2 (SARS-CoV-2) in a reverse-transcription polymerase chain reaction (RT-PCR) assay. *J Virol Method. 284*, 113926.

Hong, H., Sun, C., Wei, S., Sun, X., Mutukumira, A., Wu, X. (2020). Development of a real-time recombinase polymerase amplification assay for rapid detection of Salmonella in powdered infant formula. *Int Dairy J. 102*, 104579.

Ibrahim, S. A. E., Mohamed, S. B., Kambal, S., Diya-Aldeen, A., Ahmed, S., Faisal, B., Ismail, F., Ibrahim, A., Sabawe, A., Mohamed, O. (2020). Molecular detection of Occult Hepatitis B virus in plasma and urine of renal transplant patients in Khartoum state Sudan. *Int J Infect Dis. 97*, 126-130.

Ishige, T., Murata, S., Taniguchi, T., Miyabe, A., Kitamura, K., Kawasaki, K., Nishimura, M., Igari, H., Matsushita, K. (2020). Highly sensitive detection of SARS-CoV-2 RNA by multiplex rRT-PCR for molecular diagnosis of COVID-19 by clinical laboratories. *Clinica Chimica Acta. 507*, 139-142.

Jalandra, R., Yadav, A. K., Verma, D., Dalal, N., Sharma, M., Singh, R., Kumar, A., Solanki, P. R. (2020). Strategies and perspectives to develop SARS-CoV-2 detection methods and diagnostics. *Biomed Pharmacother. 129*, 110446.

Jaton-Ogay, K., Bille, J. (2008). Microbiological diagnosis of community-acquired respiratory tract infections by nucleic acid detection. *Expert Opin Med Diagn. 2*(8):947-961.

Javalkote, V. S., Kancharla, N., Bhadra, B., Shukla, M., Soni, B., Goodin, M., Bandyopadhyay, A., Dasgupta, S. (2020). CRISPR-based assays for rapid detection of SARS-CoV-2. *Methods*. doi: 10.1016/j.ymeth.2020.10.003.

Jung, Y. J., Park, G. S., Moon, J. H., Ku, K., Beak, S. H., Kim, S., Park, E. C., Park, D., Lee, J. H., Byeon, C. W., et al., (2020). Comparative analysis of primer-probe sets for the laboratory confirmation of SARS-CoV-2. *BioRxiv.* doi: 10.1101/2020.02.25.964775.

Kalvatchev, Z., Tsekov, I., Kalvatchev, N. (2010). Loop-mediated amplification of sensitive and specific detection of viruses. *Biotechnol Biotechnol Equip. 24*(1), 1559-1561.

Karakkat, B. B., Hockemeyer, K., Franchett, M., Olson, M., Mullenberg, C., Koch, P. L. (2018). Detection of root-infecting fungi on cool-season turfgrasses using loop-mdiated isothermal amplification and recombinase polymerase amplification. *Journal of Microbiological Methods. 151*, 90-98.

Kim, J., Jeon, S., Kim, H., et al., (2012). Multiplex real-time polymerase chain reaction-based method for the rapid detection of gyrA and parC mutations in quinolone-resistant Escherichia coli and Shigella spp. *Osong Public Health Res Perspect. 3*(2), 113-117.

Kim, W., Lee, S. H., Ahn, Y. J., Lee, S. H., Ryu, J., Choi, S. K., Choi, S. (2018). A label-free cellulose SERS biosensor chip with improvement of nanoparticle-enhanced LSPR effects for early diagnosis of subarachnoid hemorrhage-induced complications. *Biosens Bioelectron. 111*, 59-65.

Kitagawa, Y., Orihara, Y., Kawamura, R., Imai, K., Sakai, J., Tarumoto, N., Matsuoka, M., Takeuchi, S., Maesaki, S., Maeda, T. (2020). Evaluation of rapid diagnosis of novel coronavirus dieases (COVID-19) using loop-mediated isothermal amplification. *J Clin Virol. 129*, 104446.

Kost, G. J. (2018). Molecular and point-of-care diagnostics for Ebola and new threats: national POCT policy and guidelines will stop epidemics. *Expert Review of Molecular Diagnostics. 18*(7), 657-673.

Kurn, N., Chen, P., Heath, J. D., Kopf-Sill, A., Stephens, K. M., Wang, S. (2005). Novel isothermal, linear nucleic acid amplification systems for highly multiplexed application. *Clin Chem. 51*(10), 1973-1981.

Kwiatkowski, R. W., Lyamichev, V., de Arruda, M., Neri, B. (1999). Clinical, genetic and pharmacogenetic applications of the invader assay. *Mol Diagn. 4*(4), 353-364.

Lalle, E., Borxi, L., Castilletti, C., Meschi, S., Selleri, M., Carletti, F., Lapa, D., Travaglini, D., Ippolito, G., Capobianchi, M. R., Caro, A. D. (2010). Design and clinical application of a molecular method for detection and typing of influenza A/H1N1pdm virus. *Journal of Virological Methods. 163*(2), 486-488.

Lasken, R. S., Egholm, A. (2003). Whole genome amplification: abundant supplies of DNA from precious samples or clinical specimens. *Trends Biotechnol. 21*(12), 531-535.

Lee, S. H., Baek, Y. H., Kim, Y. H., et al., (2016). One-pot reverse transcriptional loop-mediated isothermal amplification (RT-LAMP) for detecting MERS-CoV. *Front Microbiol.* 7: 2166.

Lehto, M. T., Peery, H. E., Cashman, N. R. (2006). Current and future molecular diagnostics for prion diseases. *Expert Review of Molecular Diagnostics. 6*(4), 597-611.

Lemieux, B., Li, Y., Kong, H., Tang, Y. W. (2012). Near instrument-free, simple molecular device for rapid detection of herpes simplex viruses. *Expert Review of Molecular Diagnostic. 12*(5), 437-443.

Li, Y., Luo, D. (2006). Multiplexed molecular detection using encoded microparticles and nanoparticles. *Expert Review of Molecular Diagnostic. 6*(4), 567-574.

Li, Q., Yue, Z., Liu, H., Liang, C., Zheng, X., Zhao, Y., Chen, X., Xiao, X., Chen, C. (2010). Development and evaluation of a loop-mediated isothermal amplification assay for rapid detection of lymphocystis disease virus. *J Virol Methods. 163*(2), 378-384.

Li, Y., Yu, Z., Jiao, S., Liu, Y., Ni, H., Wang, Y. (2020). Development of a recombinase-aided amplification assay for rapid and sensitive detection of porcine cirvovirus 3. *Journal of Virological Methods. 282*, 113904.

Li, L., Liang, Y., Hu, F., Yan, H., Li, Y., Xie, Z., Huang, L., Zhao, J., Wan, Z., Wang, H., Shui, J., Cai, W., Tang, S. (2020). Molecular and serological characterization of SARS-CoV-2 infection among COVID-19 patients. *Virology. 551*, 26-35.

Linh, V. T. N., Moon, J., Mun, C. W., Devaraj, V., Oh, J. W., Park, S. G., Kim, D. H., Choo, J., Lee, Y. I., Jung, H.S. (2019). A facile low-cost paper-based SERS substrate for label-free molecular detection. *Sensors and Actuators: B. Chemical. 291*, 369-377.

Liotti, F. M., Menchinelli, G., Marchetti, S., Morandotti, G. A., Sanguinetti, M., Posteraro, B., Cattani, P. (2020). Evaluation the newly developed BioFire COVID-19 test for SARS-CoV-2 molecular detection. *Clinical Microbiology and Infection.* doi:10.1016/j.cmi.2020.07.026.

Little, M. C., Andrews, J., Moore, R., Bustos, S., Jones, L., Embres, C., Durmowicz, G., Harris, J., Berger, D., Yanson, K., Rostkowski, C., Yursis, D., Price, J., Fort, T., Walters, A., Collis, M., Llorin, O., Wood, J., Failing, F., O'Keefe, C., Scrivens, B., Pope, B., Hansen, T., Marino, K., Williams, K., et al., (1999). Strand displacement amplification and homogenous real-time detection incorporated in a second-generation DNA probe system, BDProbeTecET. *Clin. Chem. 45*(6 Pt 1), 777-784.

Liu, H., Wang, J., Li, P., Bai, L., Jia, J., Pan, A., Long, X., Cui, W., Tang, X. (2020). Rapid detection of P-35S and T-nos in genetically modified organisms by recombinase polymerase amplification combined with a lateral flow strip. *Food Control. 107*, 106775.

Lu, R., Wang, J., Li, M., Wang, Y., Dong, J., Cai, W. (2020). SARS-CoV-2 detection using digital PCR for COVID-19 diagnostic, treatment monitoring and criteria for discharge. *MedRxiv*. doi: 10.1101/2020.03.24.20042689.

Lubke, N., Senff, T., Scherger, S., Hauka, S., Andree, M., Adams, O., Timm, J., Walker, A. (2020). Extraction-free SARS-CoV-2 detection by rapid RT-qPCR universal for all primary respiratory materials. *Journal of Clinical Virology. 130*, 104579.

Luthra, R., Medeiros, K. J. (2004). Isothermal multiple displacement amplification: a highly reliable approach for generating unlimited high molecular weight genomic DNA from clinical specimens. *J Mol Diagn. 6*(3), 236-242.

Lv, J., Yang, J., Xue, J., Zhu, P., Liu, L., Li, S. (2020). Detection of SARS-CoV-2 RNA residue on object surfaces in nucleic acid testing laboratory using droplet digital PCR. *Science of The Total Environment. 742*, 140370.

Lv, D. F., Ying, Q. M., Weng, Y. S., Shen, C. B., Chu, J. G., Kong, J. P., Sun, D. H., Gao, X., Weng, X. B., Chen, X. Q. (2020). Dynamic change process of target genes by RT-PCR testing of SARS-CoV-2 during the course of a coronavirus disease 2019 patient. *Clinica Chimica Acta. 506, 172-175.*

Mak, G. C. K., Cheng, P. K. C., Lau, S. S. Y., Wong, K. K. Y., Lau, C. S., Lam, E. T. K., Chan, R. C. W., Tsand, D. N. C. (2020). Evaluation of rapid antigen test for detection of SARS-CoV-2 virus. *Journal of Clinical Virology. 129*, 104500.

Mangal, M., Bansal, S., Sharma, S. K., Gupta, R. K. (2016). Molecular detection of foodborne pathogens: A rapid and accurate answer to food safety. *Critical Reviews in Food Science and Nutrition. 56*(9), 1568-1584.

Menova, P., Raindlova, V., Hocek, M. (2013). Scope and limitations of the nicking enzyme amplification reaction for the synthesis of base-modified oligonucleotides and primers for PCR. *Bioconjug Chem. 24*, 1081-1093.

Metsky, H. C., Freije, C. A., Kosoko-Thoroddsen, T. S. F., Sabeti, P. C., Myhrvold, C. (2020). CRISPR-based surveillance for COVID-19 using genomically-comprehensive machine learing design. *BioRxiv*. doi: 10.1101/2020.02.26.967026.

Michel, D., Dazer, K. M., GroB, R., Conzelmann, C., Muller, J. A., Freischmidt, A., Weishaupt, J. H., Heller, S., Munch, J., Michel, M., Stamminger, T., Kleger, A., Otto, M. (2020). Rapid, convenient and efficient kit-independent detection of SARS-CoV-2 RNA. *Journal of Virological Methods. 286*, 113965.

Molenkamp, R., van der Ham, A., Schinkel, J., Beld, M. (2007). Simultaneous detection of five different DNA targets by real-time Taqman PCR using the Roche LightCycler480: Application in viral molecular diagnostics. *Journal of Virological Methods. 141*, 205-211.

Montesinos, I., Gruson, D., Kabamba, B., Dahma, H., Wijngaert, S. V. D., Reza, S., Carbone, V., Vandenberg, O., Gulbis, B., Wolff, F., Rodriguez-Villalobos, H. (2020). Evaluation of two automated and three rapid lateral flow immunoassays for the detection of anti-SARS-CoV-2 antibodies. *Journal of Clinical Virology. 128*: 104413.

Mori, Y., Notomi, T. (2009). Loop-mediated isothermal amplification (LAMP): A rapid, accurate, and cost-effective method for infectious diseases. *Journal of Infection and Chemotherapy. 15*(2), 62-69.

Mostafa, H. H., Hardick, J., Morehead, E., Miller, J. A., Gaydos, C. A., Manabe, Y. C. (2020). Comparison of the analytical sensitivity of seven commonly used commercial SARS-CoV-2 automated molecular assays. *Journal of Clinical Virology. 130*, 104578.

Mousavi, S. M., Zeinoddini, M., Azizi, A., Saeedinia, A., Monazah, A. (2017). Molecular detection of zonula occludens toxin (zot) gene in Vibrio cholera O1 using PCR. *Research in Molecular Medicine. 5*(3), 37-40.

Nakano, R., Okamoto, R., Nakano, A., et al., (2013). Rapid assay for detecting gyrA and parC mutations associated with fluoroquinolone resistance in Enterobacteriaceae. *J Microbiol Methods. 94*, 213-216.

Nelson, M. M., Waldron, C. L., Bracht, J. R. (2019). Rapid molecular detection of macrolide resistance. *BMC Infectious Diseases. 19*, 144.

Nie, S., Roth, R. B., Stiles, J., Mikhlina, A., Lu, X., Tang, Y. W., Babady, N. E. (2014). Valuation of Alere I influenza A&B for rapid detection of influenza viruses A and B. *J Clin Microbiol. 52*, 3339-3344.

Notomi, T., Okayama, H., Masubuchi, H., Yonekawa, Y., Watanabe, K., Amino, N., Hase, T. (2000). Loop-mediated isothermal amplification of DNA. *Nucleic Acids Res. 28*(12), E63.

Onseedaeng, S., Ratthawongjirakul, P. (2016). Rapid detection of genomic mutations in gyrA and parC genes of Escherichia coli by multiplex allele specific polymerase chain reaction. *J Clin Lab Anal. 30*(6), 947-955.

Packey, C. D., Shanahan, M. T., Manick, S., Bower, M. A., Ellermann, M., Tonkonogy, S. L., Carroll, I. M., Sartor, R. B. (2013). Molecular detection of bacterial contamination in gnotobiotic rodent units. *Gut Microbes. 4*(5), 361-370.

Parida, M., Posadas, G., Inoue, S., Hasebe, F., Morita, K. (2004). Real-time reverse transcription loop-mediated isotheral amplification for rapid detection of West Nile virus. *J Clin Microbiol. 42*(1), 257-263.

Park, G. S., Ku, K., Baek, S. H., Kim, S. J., Kim, S. I., Kim, B. T., Meng, J. S. (2020). Development of reverse transcription loop-mediated isothermal amplification assays targeting severe acute respiratory syndrome coronavirus 2 (SARS-CoV-2). *The Journal of Molecular Diagnostics. 22*(6), 729-735.

Peckle, M., Pires, M. S., Silva, C. B. D., Costa, R. L. D., Vitari, G. L. V., Senra, M. V. X., Dias, R. J. P., Santos, H. A., Massard, C. L. (2018). Molecular characterization of Theileria equi in horses from the state of Rio de Janeiro, Brazil. *Ticks Tick Borne Dis. 9*: 349-353.

Perchetti, G. A., Nalla, A. K., Huang, M. L., Zhu, H., Wei, Y., Stensland, L., Loprieno, M. A., Jerome, K. R., Greninger, A. L. (2020). Validatin of SARS-CoV-2 detection across multiple specimen types. *Journal of Clinical Virology. 128*, 104438.

Polstra, A. M., Goudsmit, J., Cornelissen, M. (2002). Development of real-time NASBA assays with molecular beacon detection to quantify mRNA coding for HHV-8 lytic and latent genes. *BMC Infect Dis. 2*, 18.

Porte, L., Legarraga, P., Vollrath, V., Aguilera, X., Munita, J. M., Araos, R., Pizarro, G., Vial, P., Iruretagoyena, M., Dittrich, S., Weitzel, T. (2020). Evaluation of a novel antigen-based rapid detection test for the diagnosis of SARS-CoV-2 in respiratory samples. *International Journal of Infectious Diseases. 99*, 328-333.

Poon, L. L. M., Chan, K. H., Wong, O. K., Yam, W. C., Yuen, K. Y., Guan, Y., Lo, Y. M. D., Peiris, J. S. M. (2003). Early diagnosis of SARS coronavirus infection by real time RT-PCR. *J Clin Virol. 28*(3), 233-238.

Pyrc, K., Milewska, A., Potempa, J. (2011). Development of loop-mediated isothermal amplification assay for detection of human coronavirus-NL63. *Journal of Virological Methods. 175*(1): 133-136.

Qi, J., Li, X., Zhang, Y., Shen, X., Song, G., Pan, J., Fan, T., Wang, R., Li, L., Ma, X. (2019). Development of a suplex reverse transcription recombinase-aided amplification assay for respiratory syncytial virus incorporating an internal control. *Archives of Virology. 164*, 1843-1850.

Rahimi, A., Mirzazadeh, A., Tavakolpour, S. (2020). Genetics and genomics of SARS-CoV-2: A review of the literature with the special focus on genetic diversity and SARS-CoV-2 genome detection. *Genomics*. doi: 10.1016/j.ygeno.2020.09.059.

Ramachandran, R., Muniyandi, M. (2018). Rapid molecular diagnostics for multi-drug resistance tuberculosis in India. *Expert Review of Anti-infective Therapy. 16(3), 197-204.*

Reokrungruang, P., Chatnuntawech, I., Dharakul, T., Bamrungsap, S. (2019). A simple paper-based surface enhanced Raman scattering (SERS) platform and magnetic separation for cancer screening. *Sens Actuators B Chem*. *285*:462-469.

Ribeiro, V. S. T., Raboni, S. M., Suss, P. H., Cieslinski, J., Kraft, L., dos Santos, J. S., Pereira, L., Tuon, F. F. (2019). Detection and quantification of human immunodeficiency virus and hepatitis C virus in cadaveric tissue donors using different molecular tests. *Journal of Clinical Virology*. *121*, 104203.

Rizvi, A. S., Murtaza, G., Yan, D., Irfan, M., Xue, M., Meng, Z. H. and Qu, F. (2020). Development of molecularly imprinted 2D photonic crystal hydrogel sensor for detection of L-Kynurenine in human serum. *Talanta*. *208*, 120403.

Rodel, J., Egerer, R., Suleyman, A., Sommer-Schmid, B., Baier, M., Henke, A., Edel, B., Loffler, B. (2020). Use of the variplex™ SARS-CoV-2 RT-LAMP as a praid molecular assay to complement RT-PCR for COVID-19 diagnosis. *Journal of Clinical Virology*. *132*, 104616.

Sakanashi, D., Asai, N., Nakamura, A., Miyazaki, N., Kawamoto, Y., Ohno, T., Yamada, A., Koita, I., Suematsu, H., Hagihara, M., Shiota, A., Kurumiya, A., Sakata, M., Kato, S., Muramatsu, Y., Koizumi, Y., Kishino, T., Ohashi, W., Mikamo, H. (2020). Comparative evaluation of nasopharyngeal swab and saliva specimens for the molecular detection of SARS-CoV-2 RNA in Japanese patients with COVID-19. *J Infect Chemother*. doi: 10.1016/j.jiac.2020.09.027.

Schmitt, F., Barroca, H. (2012). Role of ancillary studies in fine-needle aspiration from selected tumors. *Cancer Cytopathol*. *120*, 145-160.

Shang, Y., Sun, J., Ye, Y., Zhang, J., Zhang, Y., Sun, X. (2020). Loop-mediated isothermal amplification-based microfluidic chip for pathogen detection. *Critic Rev Food Sci Nutr*. *60*(2), 201-224.

Shen, M., Zhou, Y., Ye, J., Al-maskri, A. A. A., Kang, Y., Zeng, S., Cai, S. (2020). Recent advances and perspectives of nucleic acid detection for coronavirus. *Journal of Pharmaceutical Analysis*. *10*, 97-101.

Shi, P. Y., Kramer, L. D. (2003). Molecular detection of West Nile virus RNA. *Expert Review of Molecular Diagnostics*. *3*(3), 357-366.

Shi, L., Yu, X. W., Yao, W., Yu, B. L., He, K. K., Gao, Y., Zhang, Y. X., Tian, G. B., Ping, J. H., Wang, X. R. (2019). Development of a reverse-transcription loop-mediated isothermal amplification assay to detect avian influenza viruses in clinical specimens. *Journal of Integrative Agriculture*. *18*(7), 1428-1435.

Shirato, K., Yano, T., Senba, S., Akachi, S., Kobayashi, T., Nishinaka, T., Notomi, T., Matsuyama, S. (2014). Detection of Middle East respiratory syndrome coronavirus using reverse transcription loop-mediated isothermal amplification (RT-LAMP). *Virol J*. *11*, 139.

Shirato, K., Semba, S., El-Kafrawy, S. A., Hassan, A. M., Tolah, A. M., Takayama, I., Kageyama, T., Notomi, T., Kamitani, W., Matsuyama, S., Azhar, E. I. (2018). Development of fluorescent reverse transcription loop-mediated isothermal amplification (RT-LAMP) using quenching probes for the detection of the Middle East respiratory syndrome coronavirus. *J Virol Methods. 258*:41-48.

Singh, R., Maganti, R. J., Jabba, S. V., Wang, M., Deng, G., Heath, J. D., Kurn, N., Wangemann, P. (2005). Microarray-based comparison of three amplification methods for nanogram amounts of total RNA. *Am J Physiol Cell Physiol. 288*(5), C1179-89.

Singh, D. V. (2003). Hexaplex PCR for rapid detection of virulence factors. *Exp Rev Mol Diagn. 3*(6), 781-784.

Sohrabi, C., Alsafi, Z., O'Neill, N., Khan, M., Kerwan, A., Al-Jabir, A., Iosifidis, C., Agha, R. (2020). World Health Organization declares global emergency: a review of the 2019 novel coronavirus (COVID-19). *Int J Surg. 76*, 71-76.

Stone, C. B., Mahony, J. B. (2014). Molecular detection of bacterial and viral pathogens-Where do we go from here? *Clinical Microbiol. 3*, 6.

Sun, N., Wang, W., Wang, J., Yao, X., Chen, F., Li, X., Yinglei, Y., Chen, B. (2018). Reverse transcription recombinase polymerase amplification with lateral flow dipstikcs for detection of influenza A virus and subtyping of H1 and H3. *Mol Cell Probes. 42*, 25-31.

Taha, M. K. (2002). Molecular detection and characterization of Neisseria meningitides. *Expert Rev Mol Diagn. 2*(2), 143-150.

Takayama, I., Nakauchi, M., Takahashi, H., Oba, K., Semba, S., Kaida, A., Kubo, H., Saito, S., Nagata, S., Odagiri, T., Kageyama, T. (2019). Development of real-time fluorescent reverse transcription loop-mediated isothermal amplification assay with quenching primer for influenza virus and respiratory syncytial virus. *J Virol Method. 267*, 53-58.

Tan, X., Krel, M., Dolgov, E., Park, S., Li, X., Wu, W., Sun, Y. L., Zhang, J., Oo, M. K. K., Perlin, D. S., Fan, X. (2020). Rapid and quantitative detection of SARS-CoV-2 specific IgG for convalescent serum evaluation. *Biosens Bioelectron. 169*, 112572.

Tatipally, S., Srikantam, A., Kasetty, S., Kasetty, S. (2018). Polymerase chain reaction (PCR) as a potential point of care laboratory test for leprosy diagnosis- a systematic review. *Trop Med Infect Dis. 3*, 107.

Teklemariam, A. D., Samaddar, M., Alharbi, M. G., Al-Hindi, R. R., Bhunia, A. K. (2020). Biosensor and molecular-based methods for the detection of human coronaviruses: A review. *Mol Cell Probe. 54*, 101662.

Thi, L., Takayama, I., Binh, N. G., Phuong, T. T., Thi, V., Van, T., et al., (2020). A clinical-based direct real-time fluorescent reverse transcription loo-mediated isothermal amplification assay for influenza virus. *J Virol Method. 277*, 113801.

Tsoktouridis, G., Tsiamis, G., Koutinas, N., Mantell, S. (2014). Molecular detection of bacteria in plant tissues, using universal 16S ribosomal DNA degenerated primers. *Biotechnology and Biotechnology Equipment. 28*(4), 583-591.

Tyagi, S., Kramer, F. R. (1996). Molecular beacons: probes that fluoresce upon hybridization. *Nat Biotechnol. 14*(3), 303-308.

Tyagi, S., Bratu, D. P., Kramer, F. R. (1998). Multicolor molecular beacons for allele discrimination. *Nat Biotechnol. 16*(1), 49-53.

Uhteg, K., Jarrett, J., Richards, M., Howard, C., Morehead, E., Geahr, M., Gluck, L., Hanlon, A., Ellis, B., Kaur, H., Simner, P., Carroll, K. C., Mostafa, H. H. (2020). Comparing the analytical performance of three SARS-CoV-2 molecular diagnostic assays. *J Clin Virol. 127*, 104384.

Ulloa, S., Bravo, C., Parra, B., Ramirez, E., Acevedo, A., Fasce, R., Fernandez, J. (2020). A simple method for SARS-CoV-2 detection by rRT-PCR without the use of a commercial RNA extraction kit. *J Virol Method. 285*, 113960.

Vieria, M. I. B., Costa, M. M., de Oliveira, M. T., Goncalves, L. R., Andre, M. R., Machado, R. Z. (2018). Serological detection and molecular characterization of piroplasmids in equids in Brazil. *Acta Trop. 179*, 81-87.

Voermans, J., Deniz, S., Koopmans, M., van der Eijk, A., Pas, S. (2016). Performance of a molecular diagnostic, multicode based, sample-to-answer assay for the simultaneous detection of Influenza A,B and respiratory syncytial viruses. *J Clin Virol. 82*, S34.

Vries, E. V. D., Anber, J., Linden, A. V. D., Wu, Y., Maaskant, J., Stadhouders, R., Beek, R. V., Rimmelzwaan, G., Osterhaus, A., Boucher, C., Schutten, M. (2013). Molecular assay for quantitative and qualitative detection of influenza virus and oseltamivir resistance mutations. *J Mol Diagn. 15*(3), 347-354.

Wang, Z. H., Wang, X. J., Hou, S. H. (2019). Development of a recombinase polymerase amplification assay with lateral flow dipstick for rapid detection of feline parvovirus. *J Virol Method. 271*, 113679.

Wang, K. L, Deng, Q. Q., Chen, J. W., Shen, W. K. (2019). Development of a reverse transcription loop-mediated isothermal amplification assay for rapid and visual detection of Sugarecane streak mosaic virus in sugarcane. *Crop Prot. 119*, 38-45.

Wang, P. (2020). Combination of serological total antibody and RT-PCR test for detection of SARS-CoV-2 infection. *J Virol Method. 283*, 113919.

Wang, J., Cai, K., He, X., Shen, X., Wang, J., Liu, J., Xu, J., Qiu, F., Lei, W., Cui, L., Ge, Y., Wu, T., Zhang, Y., Yan, H., Chen, Y., Yu, J., Ma, X., Shi, H., Zhang, R., Li, X., Gao, Y., Niu, P., Tan, W., Wu, G., Jiang, Y., Xu, W., Ma, X. (2020). Multiple-centre clinical evaluation of an ultrafast single-tube assay for SARS-CoV-2 RNA. *Clin Microbiol Infect. 26*, 1076-1081.

Weile, J., Knabbe, C. (2009). Current applications and future trends of molecular diagnostics in clinical bacteriology. *Anal Bioanal Chem. 394*, 731-742.

Wharam, S. D., Marsh, P., Lloyd, J. S., Ray, T. D., Mock, G. A., Assenberg, R., McPhee, J. E., Brown, P., Weston, A., Cardy, D. L. (2001). Specific detection of DNA and RNA targets using a novel isothermal nucleic acid amplification assay based on the formation of a three way junction structure. *Nucleic Acids Res. 29*(11), E54-4.

Wu, T., Ge, Y., Zhao, K., Zhu, X., Chen, Y., Wu, B., Zhu, F., Zhu, B., Cui, L. (2020). A reverse-transcription recombinase-aided amplification assay for the rapid detection of N gene of severe acute respiratory syndrome coronavirus 2 (SARS-CoV-2). *Virology. 549*, 1-4.

Xi, Y., Xu, C. Z., Xie, Z. Z., Zhu, D. L., Dong, J. M., Xiao, G. (2019). Development of a reverse transcription recombinase polymerase amplification assay for rapid detection of human respiratory syncytial virus. *Mol Cell Probes. 45*, 8-13.

Xia, S., Chen, X. (2020). Single-copy sensitive, field-deployable and simultaneous dual-gene detection of SARS-CoV-2 RNA via modified RT-RPA. *Cell Discov. 6*, 37.

Xia, J., Tong, J., Liu, M., Shen, Y., Guo, D. (2020). Evaluation of coronavirus in tears and conjunctival secretions of patients with SARS-CoV-2 infection. *J Med Virol*. 92: 589-594.

Xing, J., Yu, J., Liu, Y. (2020). Improvement and evaluation of loop-mediated isothermal amplification combined with chromatographic flow dipstick assays for Vibrio parahaemolyticus. *J Microbiol Methods. 171*, 105866.

Xu, Y. Z., Fang, D. Z., Chen, F. F., Zhao, Q. F., Cai, C. M., Cheng, M. G. (2020). Utilization of recombinase polymerase amplification method combined with lateral flow dipstick for visual detection of respiratory syncytial virus. *Mol Cell Probe. 49*, 101473.

Yam, W. C., Chan, K. H., Chow, K. H., Poon, L. L. M., Lam, H. Y., Yuen, K. Y., Seto, W. H., Peiris, J. S. M. (2005). Clinical evaluation of real-time PCR assay for rapid diagnosis of SARS coronavirus during outbreak and post-epidemic periods. *J Clin Virol. 33*(1), 19-24.

Yan, C., Cui, J., Huang, L., Du, B., Chen, L., Xue, G., Li, S., Zhang, W., Zhao, L., Sun, Y., Yao, H., Li, N., Zhao, H., Feng, Y., Liu, S., Zhang, Q., Liu, D., Yuan, J. (2020). Rapid and visual detection of 2019 novel coronavirus (SARS-CoV-2) by a reverse transcription of loop-mediated isothermal amplification assay. *Clin Microbiol Infect. 26*(6), 773-779.

Yang, J. L., Ma, G. P., Yang, R., Yang, S. Q., Fu, L. Z., Cheng, A. C., et al., (2010). Simple and rapid detection of Salmonella serovar Enteritidis under field conditions by loop-mediated isothermal amplification. *J Appl Microbiol. 109*(5), 1715-1723.

Yang, Z., Wang, N., Wen, H., Cui, R., Yu, J., Yang, S., Qu, T., Wang, X., He, S., Qi, J., Wang, J., Ye, Q., Liu, Y. (2019). An amplification-free detection method of nucleic acids by a molecular beacon probe based on endonuclease activity. *Sensors and Actuators: B. Chemical. 298*, 126901.

Yin, P., Choi, H. M., Calvert, C. R., Pierce, N. A. (2008). Programming biomolecular self assembly pathways. *Nature. 451*(7176), 318-322.

Yu, L., Wu, S., Hao, X., Li, X., Liu, X., Ye, S., Han, H., Dong, X., Li, X., Li, J., Liu, N., Liu, J., Zhang, W., Pelechano, V., Chen, W.-H., Yin, X. (2020). Rapid colorimetric detection of COVID-19 coronavirus using a reverse trans- scriptional loop-mediated isothermal amplification (RT-LAMP) diagnostic platform: iLACO. *MedRxiv*. doi: 10.1101/2020.02.20.20025874.

Zhang, W., Li, B., Chen, L., Wang, Y., Gao, D., Ma, X., Wu, A. (2014). Brushing, a simple way to fabricate SERS active paper substrates. *Anal Methods. 6*, 2066-2071.

Zhen, W., Berry, G. J. (2020). Development of a new multiplex real time RT-PCR assay for SARS-CoV-2 detection. *J Mol Diagn*. doi: 10.1016/j.jmoldx.2020.09.004.

Zheng, L. L., Cui, J. T., Han, H. Y., Hou, H. L., Wang, L., Liu, F., Chen, H. Y. (2020). Development of a duplex SYBR GreenI based real-time PCR assay for detection of porcine epidemic diarrhea virus and porcine bocavirus3/4/5. *Mol Cell Probes. 51*, 101544.

Zhu, X., Wang, X., Han, L., Chen, T., Wang, L., Li, H., Li, S., He, L., Fu, X., Chen, S., Xing, M., Chen, H., Wang, Y. (2020). Multiplex reverse transcription loop-mediated isothermal amplification combined with nanoparticle-based lateral flow biosensor for the diagnosis of COVID-19. *Biosens Bioelectron. 166*, 112437.

Zhu, X., Wang, X., Han, L., Chen, T., Wang, L., Li, H., Li, S., He, L., Fu, X., Chen, S., et al., (2020). Reverse transcription loop-mediated isothermal amplification combined with nanoparticles-based biosensor for diagnosis of COVID-19. *MedRxiv*. doi: 10.1101/2020.03.17.20037796.

Zou, J., Zhi, S., Chen, M., Sun, X., Kang, L., Li, C., Su, X., Zhang, S., Ge, S., Li, W. (2020). Heat inactivation decreased the qualitative real-time RT-PCR detection rates of clinical samples with high cycle threshold values in COVID-19. *Diagn Microbiol Infect Dis*. *98*, 115109.

About the Authors

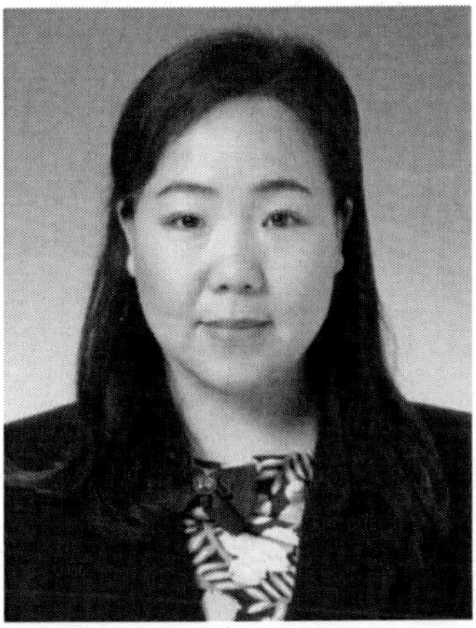

Wenli Sun
Biotechnology Research Institute,
Chinese Academy of Agricultural
Sciences,
Beijing, China

She is an associate professor working on traditional Chinese medicine, allelopathic influence and sustainable agriculture. She is also working on topics which are related to Biotechnology and Molecular Science. Her current research is a survey on the history of human coronavirus and the influence of traditional Chinese medicine in prevention and treatment of human coronavirus. Her full profile is available at http://orcid.org/0000-0002-1705-2996. Corresponding Author's Email: sunwenli@caas.cn

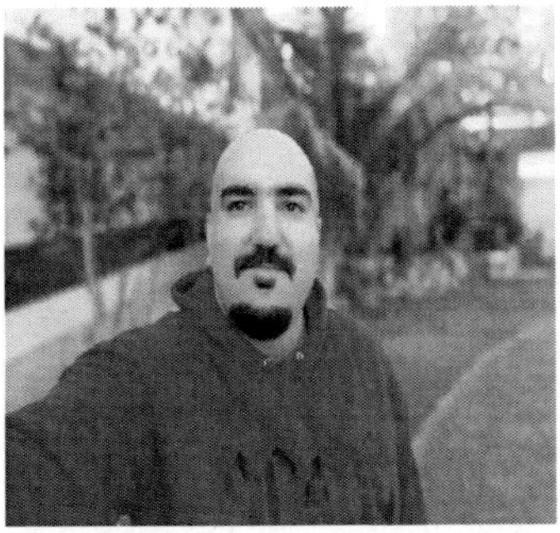

Mohamad Hesam Shahrajabian
Biotechnology Research Institute,
Chinese Academy of Agricultural Sciences,
Beijing, China

He is a senior researcher of Agronomy and Biotechnology. He is interested in crops and herbs which are related to traditional Medicine, especially Chinese and Iranian traditional Medicine crops relating to organic farming and sustainable agriculture. His current research is on the influence of medicinal herbs and fruits on human coronaviruses. His full profile is available at http://orcid.org/0000-0002-8638-1312. Corresponding Author's Email: hesamshahrajabian@gmail.com

Index

E

F

G

H

I

K

L

M

N

O

P

Q

R

S

T

V

Y

Z